LIMBAL RELAXING INCISIONS

A PRACTICAL GUIDE

LIMBAL RELAXING INCISIONS

A PRACTICAL GUIDE

Editor

Louis D. "Skip" Nichamin, MD

Medical Director and Managing Partner

Laurel Eye Clinic

Brookville, Pennsylvania

Associate Editor

Parag D. Parekh, MD, MPA

Laurel Eye Clinic

Brookville, Pennsylvania

CRC Press
Taylor & Francis Group
Boca Raton London New York

CRC Press is an imprint of the
Taylor & Francis Group, an **informa** business

A version of Chapter 3 has been previously published in Tasman W, Jaeger EA, eds. *Duane's Ophthalmology 2011*. Philadelphia, PA: Lippincott Williams & Wilkins; 2011.

First published 2014 by SLACK Incorporated

Published 2024 by CRC Press
2385 NW Executive Center Drive, Suite 320, Boca Raton FL 33431

and by CRC Press
4 Park Square, Milton Park, Abingdon, Oxon, OX14 4RN

CRC Press is an imprint of Taylor & Francis Group, LLC

Library of Congress Cataloging-in-Publication Data

Limbal relaxing incisions : a practical guide / [edited by] Louis D. "Skip" Nichamin.
p. ; cm.
Includes bibliographical references and index.
ISBN 978-1-61711-838-8 (alk. paper)
I. Nichamin, Louis D., editor of compilation.
[DNLM: 1. Astigmatism--surgery. 2. Refractive Surgical Procedures--methods. 3. Cornea--surgery. WW 340]
RE932
617.7'55--dc23

2014000479

ISBN: 9781617118388 (pbk)
ISBN: 9781003524847 (ebk)

DOI: 10.1201/9781003524847

Dedication

To my wife, Wendy, and sons, Alex and Sam, who have sacrificed immeasurably to allow me to pursue my professional goals and, more importantly, whose love and personal support cannot be described in the printed word.

Louis D. "Skip" Nichamin, MD

Contents

Acknowledgments

I thank my personal assistant, Georgann Null, for her 25 years of dedicated effort in helping to prepare manuscripts, presentations, clinical studies, and every other task that one could ask of their "right hand." Her degree of alacrity and pleasant nature are unsurpassed.

Louis D. "Skip" Nichamin, MD

About the Editor

Louis D. "Skip" Nichamin, MD is the Medical Director and Managing Partner of the Laurel Eye Clinic in Brookville, Pennsylvania, one of the leading private ophthalmic practices in the country. After graduating from the University of Michigan in Ann Arbor, Michigan and Wayne State University School of Medicine in Detroit, Michigan with high distinction and recognition, including membership in the Alpha Omega Alpha Honor Society, he completed his ophthalmic residency at the Sinai Hospital of Detroit in Michigan where he was awarded the H. Saul Sugar award for his outstanding performance.

Dr. Nichamin has since been the recipient of numerous awards, lectured extensively around the world, and authored hundreds of articles and chapters in the fields of cataract and refractive surgery. His broad surgical experience numbers in the tens of thousands of surgical cases and includes posterior, as well as anterior, segment procedures.

Dr. Nichamin has been a representative for the American Academy of Ophthalmology Board of Councilors and served as the Chairman of the Cataract Clinical Committee of the American Society of Cataract and Refractive Surgery. He holds a board position on the ASCRS Philanthropic Foundation. Dr. Nichamin is a committee member of the American Academy of Ophthalmology Preferred Practice Patterns and founding member of the American College of Ophthalmic Surgery. He has been awarded the Senior Achievement and Secretariat Awards by the American Academy of Ophthalmology. He is an active consultant in the ophthalmic industry and serves on numerous medical advisory boards.

About the Associate Editor

Parag D. Parekh, MD, MPA is an ophthalmologist at the Laurel Eye Clinic in Brookville, Pennsylvania, specializing in cataract and refractive surgery.

Dr. Parekh earned his college degree from Johns Hopkins University in Baltimore, Maryland and his medical degree from the University of Pennsylvania School of Medicine in Philadelphia, Pennsylvania. He was then awarded the Kennedy Fellowship to attend Harvard's John F. Kennedy School of Government in Cambridge, Massachusetts, where he earned a Master's degree studying U.S. Health Policy, Economics, and Management.

Dr. Parekh completed his residency at the Johns Hopkins Wilmer Eye Institute in Baltimore. He then specialized in cataract surgery, glaucoma surgery, cornea surgery, and LASIK during his fellowship with Minnesota Eye Consultants in Minneapolis.

Dr. Parekh is an active member of the American Academy of Ophthalmology, the American Society of Cataract & Refractive Surgery, the Vanguard Ophthalmology Society, as well as the American Medical Association. He has performed significant clinical research and written numerous scientific articles and textbook chapters. He has also won numerous awards including the Johns Hopkins Wilmer Eye Institute W. Richard Green Teaching Award, the American Medical Association Foundation Leadership Award, and the American Academy of Ophthalmology Achievement Award.

Contributing Authors

Noel A. Alpins, MD, FACS (Chapter 2)
Medical Director
NewVision Clinics
Developer
ASSORT Surgical Management Systems
Clinical Senior Lecturer
Department of Ophthalmology
Melbourne University
Cheltenham, Victoria, Australia

Allon Barsam, MD, MA, FRCOphth (Chapter 7)
Consultant Ophthalmic Surgeon
Luton and Dunstable University Hospital
Luton, Bedfordshire, United Kingdom
Focus Clinics
London, United Kingdom

Eric D. Donnenfeld, MD (Chapter 7)
Clinical Professor of Ophthalmology
New York University Medical Center
New York, New York

James P. Gills, MD (Chapter 4)
St. Luke's Cataract and Laser Institute
Tarpon Springs, Florida

Pit Gills, MD (Chapter 4)
St. Luke's Cataract and Laser Institute
Tarpon Springs, Florida

David R. Hardten, MD (Chapters 1, 5)
Minnesota Eye Consultants
Minneapolis, Minnesota

Christian C. Hester, MD (Chapter 4)
Cornea, Refractive, and Anterior Segment Surgery Fellow
Department of Ophthalmology
Baylor College of Medicine
Houston, Texas

Richard S. Hoffman, MD (Chapter 4)
Clinical Associate Professor of Ophthalmology
Casey Eye Institute
Oregon Health and Science University
Eugene, Oregon

Douglas D. Koch, MD (Chapter 4)
Professor and Allen, Mosbacher, and Law Chair in Ophthalmology
Cullen Eye Institute
Baylor College of Medicine
Houston, Texas

Richard L. Lindstrom, MD (Chapter 1)
Minnesota Eye Consultants
Minneapolis, Minnesota

Molly McDonald, OD (Chapter 1, 5)
Minnesota Eye Consultants
Minneapolis, Minnesota

Randall J. Olson, MD (Chapter 4)
Professor and Chair
Department of Ophthalmology and Visual Sciences
University of Utah
CEO
John A. Moran Eye Center
Salt Lake City, Utah

Jonathan B. Rubenstein, MD (Chapter 4)
Deutsch Family Professor
Vice-Chairman of the Department of Ophthalmology
Rush University Medical Center
Chicago, Illinois

George Stamatelatos, OD (Chapter 2)
Senior Optometrist
NewVision Clinics
Clinical Director
ASSORT Surgical Management Systems
Cheltenham, Victoria, Australia

Spencer P. Thornton, MD, FACS (Chapter 1)
Clinical Professor of Ophthalmology
Department of Ophthalmology
University of Tennessee Health Science Center
Memphis, Tennessee

R. Bruce Wallace III, MD (Chapter 4)
Clinical Director of Ophthalmology
Tulane Medical School
New Orleans, Louisiana
Clinical Director of Ophthalmology
LSU School of Medicine
New Orleans, Louisiana
Medical Director
Wallace Eye Surgery & Wallace Laser & Surgery Center
Alexandria, Louisiana

An Vo, MD (Chapter 7)
Resident in Ophthalmology
New York Medical College
Jamaica Hospital Medical Center
Queens, New York

Preface

This text is designed to serve as a succinct treatise that will provide the aspiring refractive implant surgeon with a practical guide from which they can easily incorporate incisional astigmatism surgery into their repertoire. At the same time, it offers practical pearls that the more experienced practitioner may utilize to refine his or her astigmatic refractive outcomes following lens-based surgery.

Introduction

The goal of this book is to provide readers with a concise guide of how to incorporate limbal relaxing incisions (LRIs) into their lens-based ophthalmic surgical practice. The concept of managing astigmatism at the time of cataract and implant surgery was first proposed nearly 30 years ago, but it was slow to gain favor and interest.[1-3] As cataract and implant incisions diminished in size and intraocular lens (IOL) calculations were refined, the notion of *refractive* cataract surgery began to gain credence. A recent impetus for the anterior segment surgeon to further embrace this philosophy—and to acquire the skills necessary to perform this type of lenticular refractive surgery—has been the refinement and increased use of presbyopia-correcting IOLs.[4] Indeed, there is a growing population of (older) patients seeking refractive surgery who are often better served by a lens-based procedure, rather than that of keratorefractive laser surgery.

During the mid- to late 1980s and into the 1990s, a relatively small number of avant-garde surgeons began to use astigmatic keratotomy to address pre-existing astigmatism in their cataract patients. These innovators, a number of whom are contributors to this book, did not, however, find that many of their colleagues joined their ranks, and adoption of this technique was limited. It was not until these incisions were moved more peripherally—toward the limbus, thereby making them technically more forgiving—that their popularity began to grow. Today, although the availability and increased use of toric IOLs offers an alternative to incisional surgery, LRIs remain an indispensable tool to the modern anterior segment surgeon. With the arrival of femtosecond laser-assisted cataract surgery, the need to understand the planning, use, and execution of manual relaxing incisions has never been more pressing.

This text will begin with a discussion of the history, background, and future of astigmatism management by the pioneering surgeons, Drs. Spencer Thornton and Dick Lindstrom. We will then delve into the important and sometimes confusing subject of measuring cylinder and the strategic planning for the surgical correction of astigmatism, as presented by Dr. Noel Alpins. I will then detail my personal approach to the use of LRIs, followed by 8 of the world's leading surgeons who describe in succinct fashion their technique for performing LRIs. Each of these authors will provide simple and practical clinical pearls for both the novice and experienced practitioner, with the intent that the reader will come away with a sense that he or she had just spent a morning in the operating room observing these superb teachers, gleaning the various nuances to their respective techniques. As is so commonly the case with surgical technique, one learns quickly that there is no one perfect way to "skin the proverbial cat."

Even the most highly skilled surgeon will, on occasion, miss his or her refractive mark, thus Dr. David Hardten will share approaches for astigmatic enhancement surgery. Dr. Parag Parekh will then discuss the important subject of potential complications, and finally, one of the early adopters of femtosecond laser-assisted cataract surgery and a skilled astigmatism surgeon, Dr. Eric Donnenfeld, will provide insight into the use of this important laser technology to further refine and automate astigmatism correction.

The purpose of this text is to usher the novice surgeon into the world of incisional astigmatic surgery and to provide the more experienced clinician with a means by which to refine his or her refractive result. Ultimately, we appreciate that for both surgeon and patient alike, the success of modern implant surgery is increasingly judged by our refractive and astigmatic outcomes.

Louis D. "Skip" Nichamin, MD

References

1. Osher RH. Combining phacoemulsification with corneal relaxing incisions for reduction of preexisting astigmatism. Paper presented at: Annual meeting of the American Intraocular Implant Society; 1984; Los Angeles, CA.
2. Maloney WF. Refractive cataract replacement: a comprehensive approach to maximize refractive benefits of cataract extraction. Paper presented at: the Annual meeting of the American Society of Cataract and Refractive Surgery; 1986; Los Angeles, CA.
3. Osher RH. Transverse astigmatic keratotomy combined with cataract surgery. In: Thompson K, Waring G, eds. *Contemporary Refractive Surgery-Ophthalmology Clinics of North America*. Philadelphia, PA: W.B. Saunders Co; 1992:717-725.
4. Wallace RB. *Refractive Cataract Surgery and Multifocal IOLs*. Thorofare, NJ: SLACK Incorporated; 2001.

1

History, Background, and Future of Incisional Astigmatic Surgery

Section 1: The Foundation and Future of Astigmatic Keratotomy

Spencer P. Thornton, MD, FACS

Modification and control of astigmatism has been a long-term goal of ophthalmology and is a great concern of the cataract surgeon. Despite the use of small incisions, better wound closure, and other technical improvements in cataract and corneal surgery, astigmatism has remained a problem for the cataract and refractive surgeon. Both pre-existing and postoperative astigmatism are of concern because, despite best efforts, significant amounts of astigmatism sometimes remain or develop after surgery. The clinician must then decide on whether to correct it at all and what approach should be used.

Significant amounts of astigmatism can be visually disabling, with reduction in visual acuity and symptoms such as glare, monocular diplopia, asthenopia, and distortion. Even when corrected with spectacles, astigmatism may cause off-axis blur, eye strain, glare, and visual field restriction.

Not all astigmatism needs to be corrected. Astigmatic keratotomy is not indicated if the patient is asymptomatic or if satisfactory correction can be obtained with spectacles.

The use of corneal relaxing incisions for pre-existing astigmatism at the time of cataract surgery was introduced in the 1980s by Drs. Thornton, Osher, Gills, and Nichamin, among others. In the early days of radial keratotomy (RK) and astigmatic keratotomy (AK), there was a great deal of controversy regarding whether refractive error justified surgical intervention, especially whether the pristine cornea should be altered through the use of incisions. As such, addressing astigmatism at the time of cataract surgery remained a debatable and controversial subject for many years.

It was only after early leaders in ophthalmology demonstrated the efficacy of AK, especially the safety of more peripherally located limbal relaxing incisions (LRIs), that this technique came to be accepted and more broadly utilized. New devices and instruments were needed and were subsequently developed to measure and mark for incision placement, and new knives were designed for the precise creation of these refractive incisions.

Those of us who developed these new techniques were lumped into the "buccaneer surgeon" basket. Only when these methods proved successful were we joined by other early adapters. At

Nichamin LD.
Limbal Relaxing Incisions: A Practical Guide (pp 1-13).

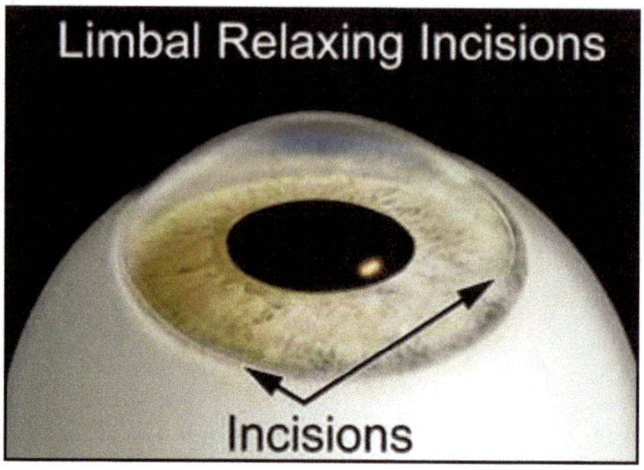

Figure 1-1. LRIs. Note placement is just inside of the true anatomic limbus.

first, what was called "experimental" and "dangerous" ultimately became mainstream and standard care.

LRIs are a modification of AK, a procedure to correct astigmatism. LRIs, however, are incisions that are placed on the far peripheral aspect of the cornea (actually just inside of the true limbus), rather than directly on the main cornea itself (as in AK), which ultimately results in a cornea that is more spherical. The astigmatism is thus reduced, and uncorrected vision is improved. Unlike AK, LRIs do not result in glare, starburst, or a weakened cornea, and the incisions heal rapidly with a rare adverse effect on the eye (Figure 1-1).

The procedure can be completed within a few minutes after numbing the eye with anesthetic drops. There is generally little, if any, postoperative discomfort. In addition, the cornea is usually stable within 2 to 4 weeks postoperatively, indicating that visual fluctuations have typically resolved by that time.

LRIs have gained widespread acceptance among cataract surgeons when the procedure is combined with cataract surgery to reduce pre-existing astigmatism. This results in improved uncorrected visual acuity postoperatively and reduced dependence on corrective eyewear.

Background

All incisions relax tissue, and all incisions have their action at right angles to the direction of the incision. Unless closed by suturing, corneal incisions act as if tissue is added (Figure 1-2).

The term *circumferential* is often confused with *transverse*. On a globe or domed surface, transverse lines are latitudinal (ie, they are parallel to the equator). Radial lines are circumferential or longitudinal (ie, they radiate out from the center of the dome around its circumference). As such, it is helpful to think of the center of the visual axis as the North Pole (Figure 1-3).

A meridian is a line (a great circle) on the surface of the globe that crosses the equator and passes through the poles, which is numbered according to degrees of longitude (eg, 80 degrees, 100 degrees, and so forth).

With-the-rule astigmatism is steeper in the vertical, or 90-degree, meridian. Against-the-rule astigmatism is steeper in the horizontal, or 180-degree, meridian.

Coupling

When an incision is placed on the surface of a dome (eg, the cornea), the relaxation or flattening of the surface occurs at right angles to the direction of the incision. Incisions that relax and flatten the steeper meridian tend to steepen the flatter meridian 90 degrees away from the direction of the incision. This change, induced 90 degrees away from a primary curvature, is termed *coupling*. The

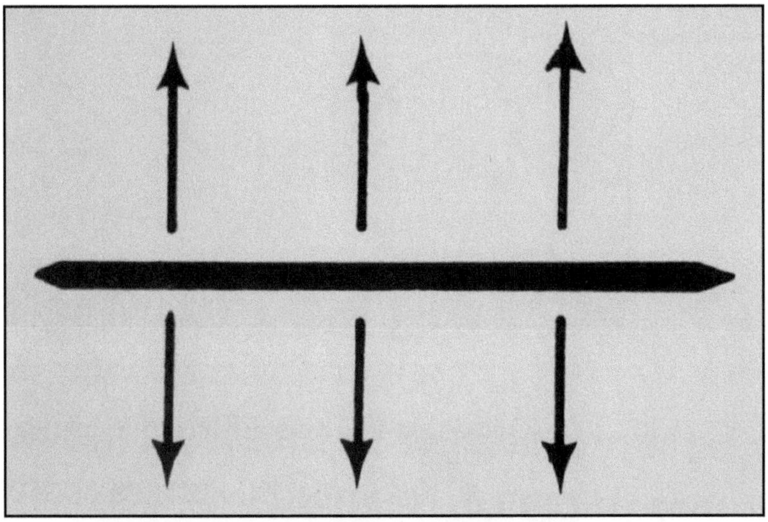

Figure 1-2. Expansion (relaxation) is always at a right angle to the direction of the incision.

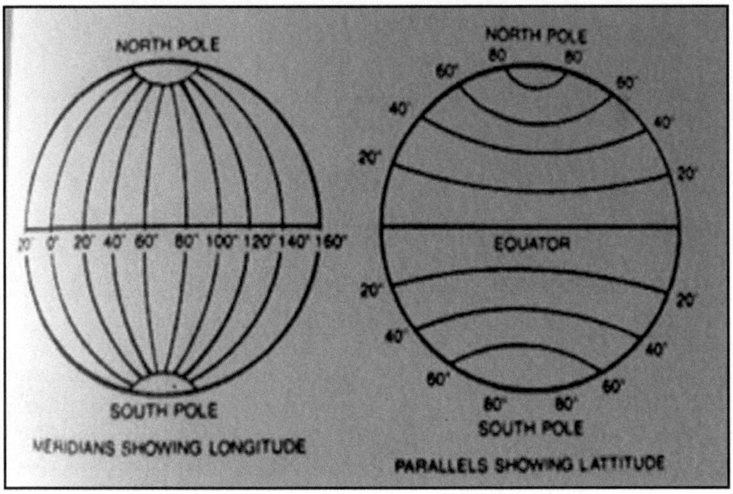

Figure 1-3. It is helpful to think of the visual axis as the North Pole and the meridian upon which relaxing incisions are centered as being a longitudinal line. Relaxing incisions are latitudinal in nature.

total amount of astigmatism corrected is equal to the sum of the change that takes place between the primary and secondary meridians (Figure 1-4).

Gauss' law (the law of elastic domes) states that for every change in curvature in one meridian, there is an equal and opposite change 90 degrees away. This can be demonstrated by squeezing a balloon or hollow rubber ball, thus steepening one meridian while flattening the other. This law assumes that the circumference of the elastic dome is unchanged, and, although it may apply to a rubber ball or a cadaver cornea, it does not apply to the living cornea after an incision has been made, as full coupling can occur only when the circumference remains the same. To understand this, we must apply what can be referred to as *the law of the modified living elastic dome* (the law of the incised cornea). This law is as follows: "The change in curvature 90 degrees away from a corneal incision is proportional to the change in the primary meridian reduced by the increase in circumference."

Radial incisions increase the radius of curvature circumferentially, flattening the central cornea indirectly by stretching because of the increased corneal circumference (Figure 1-5).

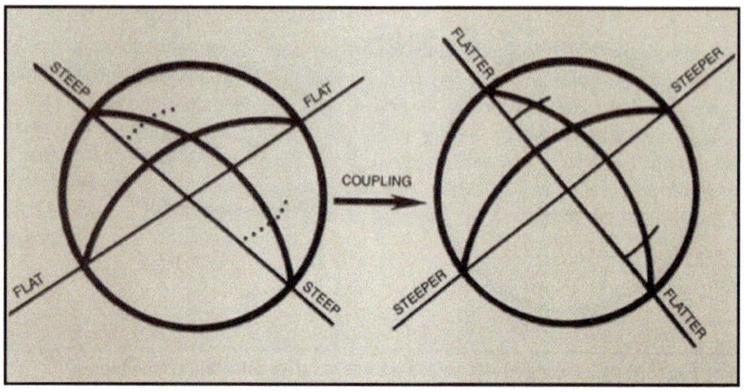

Figure 1-4. Coupling: steepening of the cornea 90 degrees away from inverse relaxing incisions.

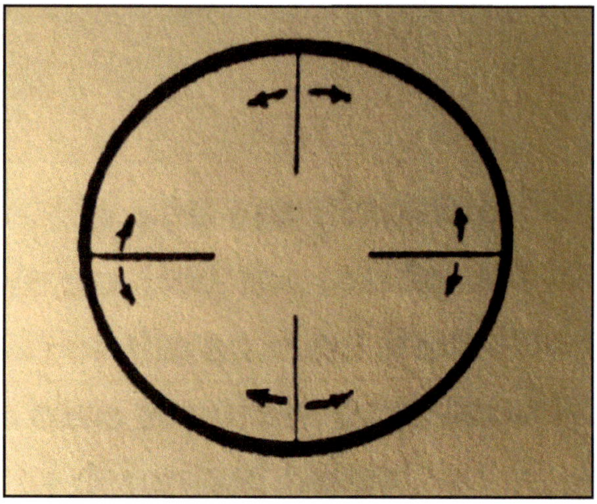

Figure 1-5. Radial incisions increase the radius circumferentially.

Adding tissue to a dome increases the radius of curvature, thus flattening the dome and decreasing the refractive power. Removing tissue from a dome reduces the radius of curvature, which steepens and increases the refractive power. Incisions in the cornea act as if tissue is added, thus increasing the radius of curvature in that meridian. As previously noted, the radius of curvature is always increased at right angles to the incision.

Transverse incisions increase the radius of curvature latitudinally; that is, parallel to the equator and in that meridian only. In contrast to radial incisions, there is no increase in circumference with transverse incisions (Figure 1-6). On the other hand, transverse incisions flatten the central cornea directly by increasing the radius of curvature in the meridian that includes the central cornea (Figure 1-7).

Laser Incisions

When laser in situ keratomileusis (LASIK) and excimer laser technology was evolving, laser-created incisions were introduced in the 1990s. Although there was some belief that this presented an advantage of precision, with minimal disturbance of corneal architecture, it was not borne out over time, and little, if any, difference in outcomes were noted. Attention was then turned to further refinement of manual incisions, with an emphasis placed on prelimbal rather than limbal incisions. Now, with the advent of femtosecond laser technology, there is a marked return of interest for this more automated approach to incision creation (see Chapter 7).

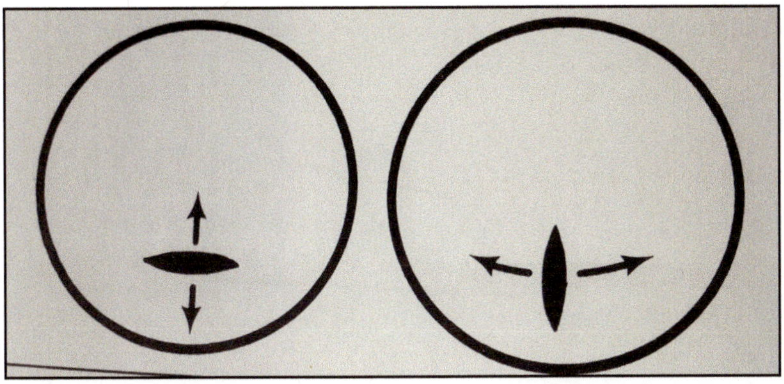

Figure 1-6. Relaxing incisions act as if tissue is added, and the radius of curvature is increased at right angles to the incision.

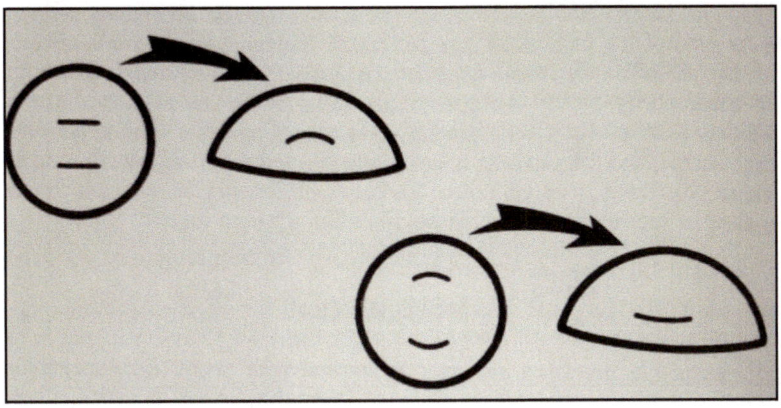

Figure 1-7. Incisions on a spherical surface appear straight or curved depending on perspective.

New Techniques

Prelimbal LRIs were introduced in the 1990s, with emphasis placed on accurate preoperative measurement of astigmatism axis and the effect of the cataract incision. Most surgeons use the standard 90% depth for incisions; however, several surgeons advocate full-thickness, penetrating incisions to address pre-existing astigmatism, such as the full-thickness astigmatic incision technique by Darrell Williams and the opposite clear corneal incision technique of Lever and Dahan.[1] Dr. Richard Mackool advocates an approach that he refers to as *double-penetrating LRIs*.[2]

The Future: Femtosecond Laser Technology and Collagen Cross-Linking to Stabilize Effect

The two most exciting areas in incisional refractive surgery appear to be in the fields of femtosecond laser technology (see Chapter 7) and corneal collagen cross-linking (CXL). The possibility of stabilizing progressive postincisional corneal changes, such as those of RK and post-LASIK ectasia, has led to increased interest in corneal CXL. Several experts have postulated that if CXL had been available during the height of interest in incisional correction of myopia and astigmatism, RK would still be the procedure of choice because corneal changes can be stabilized effectively by the use of riboflavin and ultraviolet A (UVA) light CXL.

The CXL of collagen refers to the ability of collagen fibrils to form strong chemical bonds with adjacent fibrils. Some of this naturally occurs in the cornea with aging (as well as in other parts of the body), but for immediate therapeutic effect, chemical agents (UVA light–activated

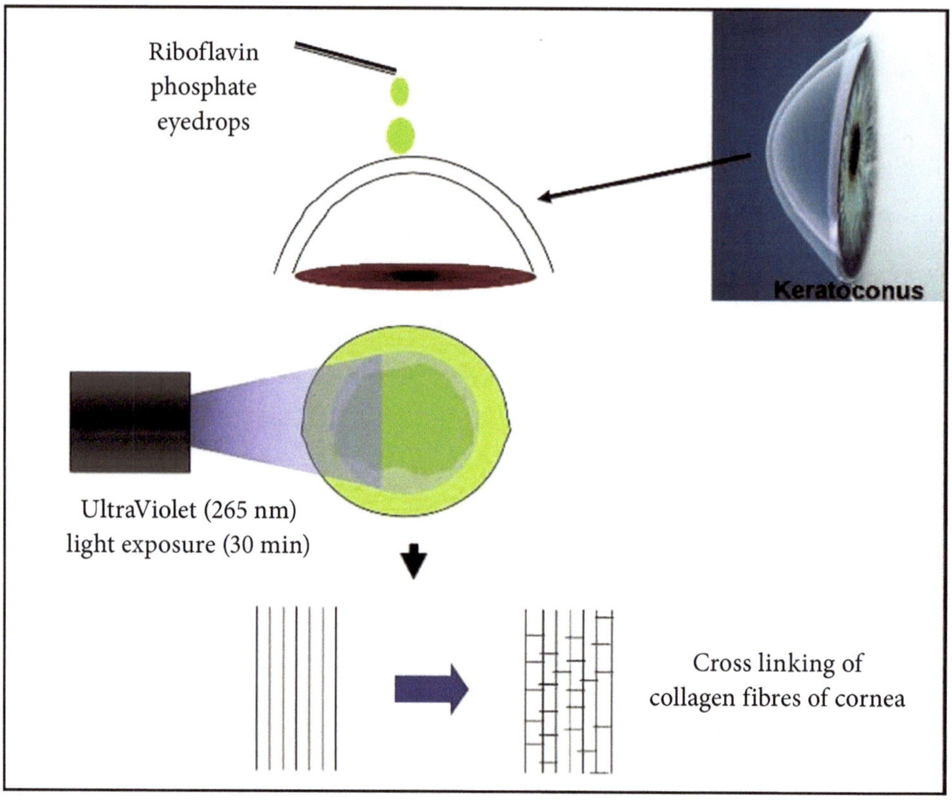

Figure 1-8. The basic principle of cross linking.

riboflavin) are used. In practice, the cornea is saturated with riboflavin, and then it is illuminated with UVA light at a frequency of 365 nm, which is a wavelength that is strongly absorbed by the riboflavin. The riboflavin has a dual action of producing free radicals, which cause CXL of the stromal collagen, thus creating stable bridges between collagen molecules, reinforcing the corneal structure, strengthening the cornea, and acting as a shield to prevent significant levels of UVA from penetrating deeper into the eye (Figure 1-8).

The photosensitizer, riboflavin, and UV light irradiance lead to strengthening of corneal tissue by increasing the collagen covalent bonds, such as in the photopolymerization in polymers, leading to a significant increase in collagen fiber diameter and reduced elasticity.

Immunofluorescent confocal microscopy has shown a pronounced compacting of collagen fibers in the anterior corneal stroma after riboflavin and UVA light exposure (Figure 1-9).

Incisional astigmatism correction—although slow to evolve and gain popularity—offers today's refractive cataract surgeon a safe and effective way of decreasing a patient's pre-existing astigmatism, thereby permitting a better visual outcome. Along with emerging laser technologies and techniques, such as CXL, to better stabilize long-term results, patients will undoubtedly continue to benefit by increasingly better refractive outcomes following lens-based surgery.

References

1. Lever J, Dahan E. Opposite clear corneal incisions to correct preexisting astigmatism in cataract surgery. *J Cataract Refract Surg.* 2000;26(6):803-805.
2. Nichamin LD, Mackool R, Donnenfeld ED. Reducing preexisting corneal astigmatism. *EyeWorld.* June 2011.

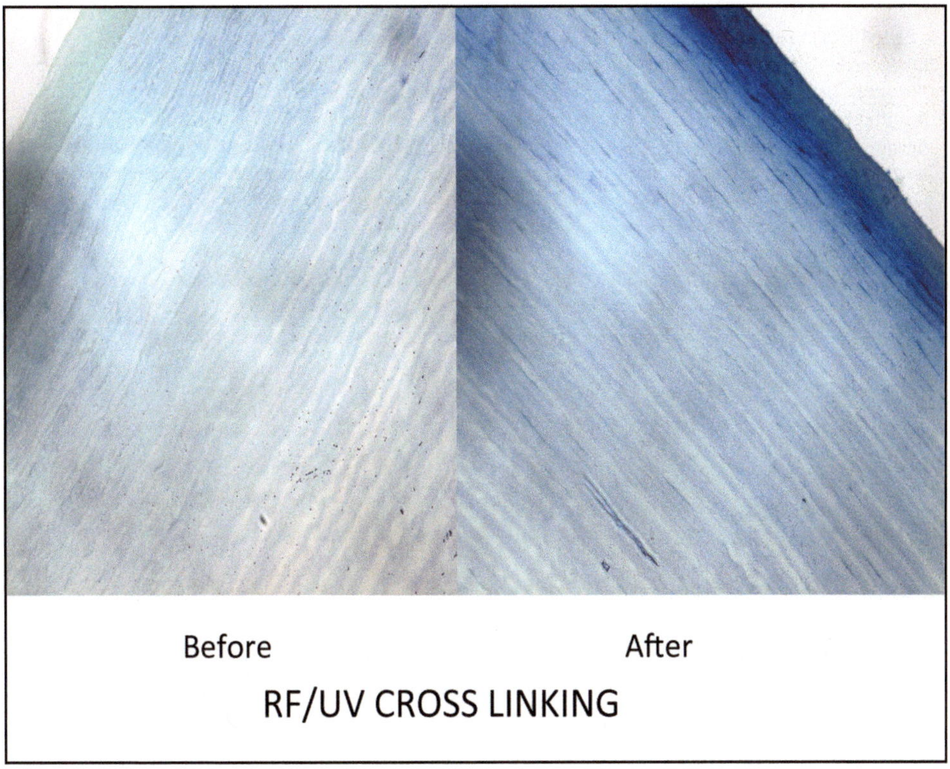

Figure 1-9. Corneal stroma before and after cross-linking. (magnification x200.)

Suggested Readings

Asri D, Touboul D, Fournié P, et al. Corneal collagen cross-linking in progressive keratoconus: multicenter results from French National Reference Center for Keratoconus. *J Cataract Refract Surg.* 2011;37(12):2137-2143.

Filippello M, Stagni E, O'Brart D. Transepithelial corneal collagen crosslinking: bilateral study. *J Cataract Refract Surg.* 2012;38(2):283-291.

Fyodorov SN, Durnev VV. Surgical correction of complicated myopic astigmatism by means of dissection of circular ligament of cornea. *Ann Ophthalmol.* 1981;13(1):115-118.

Fyodorov SN. Surgical correction of myopia and astigmatism. In: Schachar RA, Levy NS, Schachar L, eds. *Proceedings of the Keratorefractive Society.* New York, NY: LAL Publishing; 1980.

Greenstein SA, Fry KL, Hersh, MJ, Hersh PS. Higher-order aberrations after corneal collagen crosslinking for keratoconus and corneal ectasia. *J Cataract Refract Surg.* 2012;38(2):292-302.

Lindstrom RL. Minimally invasive radial keratotomy: mini-RK. *J Cataract Refract Surg.* 1995;21(1):27-34.

Nichamin LD, Thornton SP. Refining AK may enhance your cataract procedure. *Ocular Surgery News.* July 15, 1993;81-82.

Schnitzler E, Spörl E, Seiler T. Irradiation of cornea with ultraviolet light and riboflavin administration as a new treatment for erosive corneal processes: preliminary results in four patients [German]. *Klin Monatsbl Augenheilkd.* 2000;217(3):190-193.

Stein R, Stein R. Corneal collagen crosslinking: a major breakthrough in the management of keratoconus, pellucid marginal degeneration, and ectasia after LASIK. *Ophth Rounds.* 2011;9:1.

Stojanovic A, Zhang J, Chen X, Nitter TA, Chen S, Wang O. Topography-guided transepithelial surface ablation. *J Refract Surg.* 2010;26(2):145-152.

Thornton Nomogram for astigmatic keratotomy [Scientific Insert]. *ISRK Newsletter.* 1993;1(3).

Thornton SP. Astigmatic keratotomy: a review of basic concepts with case reports. *J Cataract Refract Surg.* 1990;16(4);430-435.

Thornton SP. Astigmatic keratotomy with cataract extraction: Thornton nomograms for quantitative surgery. In: Gills JP, Sanders DS, eds. *Small Incision Cataract Surgery.* Thorofare, NJ: SLACK Incorporated; 1991.
Thornton SP. Comparison of one-stage radial keratotomy with two-stage radial keratotomy in myopia (brief report). *Refract Corneal Surg.* 1989;5(1):43-45.
Thornton SP. Correction of astigmatism after cataract surgery. *Refract Corneal Surg.* 1990;6(2):131-136.
Thornton SP. One- vs two-stage procedure [Letter to the Editor]. *Refract Corneal Surg.* 1989;5(2):125.
Thornton SP. Postoperative astigmatism and its management. In: Weinstock FJ, ed. *Management and Care of the Cataract Patient.* Boston, MA: Blackwell Scientific Publications; 1992.
Thornton SP, Sanders DR. Graded nonintersecting transverse incisions for correction of idiopathic astigmatism. *J Cataract Refract Surg.* 1985;13(1):27-31.
Thornton S. Thornton guide for radial keratotomy incisions and optical zone size. *J Refract Surg.* 1985;1(1):29-33.
Vinciguerra P, Camesasca F, Albe E, Trazza S. Corneal collagen cross-linking for ectasia after excimer laser refractive surgery: 1-year results. *J Refract Surg.* 2010;26(7):486-497.

Section 2: Limbal Relaxing Incisions: History, Current State of the Art, and Future

Richard L. Lindstrom, MD; Molly McDonald, OD; and David R. Hardten, MD

Naturally occurring astigmatism is common, with up to 95% of eyes having some clinically detectable astigmatism in their refractive error.[1,2] Approximately 44% of the general population has more than 0.50 diopters (D) of astigmatism, 10% has more than 1.00 D, and 8% has 1.50 D or more.[1,3] Even with 0.50 D of astigmatism, patients perceive a blur to their vision. Astigmatism decreases visual acuity, as does myopia and hyperopia, but it is more complex in that it has both magnitude and orientation. Thus, historically, astigmatism has been more difficult to correct using spectacles, contact lenses, intraocular lenses (IOLs), or refractive surgery.[4]

Multiple names have been used to describe various incisions for the correction of astigmatism. Incisions can be straight, transverse, arcuate, or semiradial, or those associated with AK or LRIs, for the reduction of astigmatism but some general principles apply to all incisional patterns.[5] Generally, more central and longer corneal incisions create more effect, but they are also more dependent on pachymetry and are more likely to result in overcorrection and irregular astigmatism. More central incisions have been called *AK incisions*, whereas more peripheral incisions have been termed *LRIs*. In this chapter, we will refer to AK as a more general term for central corneal incisions.[6]

History of Astigmatic Keratotomy

AK appears to have been the first refractive corneal procedure performed by ophthalmologists. In 1885, Schiotz,[7] a Norwegian ophthalmologist, reported the case history of a patient who developed 19.50 D of astigmatism after cataract surgery. Four months postoperatively, he used a von Graefe knife to make a 3.5-mm penetrating incision at the limbus in the steep meridian, which reduced the astigmatism to 7.00 D. A Dutch ophthalmologist, Faber,[8] later performed perforating anterior transverse incisions in a 19-year-old patient, which reduced the patient's astigmatism from 1.50 to 0.75 D. Lucciola of Italy was the first surgeon to use nonperforating incisions to correct astigmatism.[9]

In 1894, Bates[10] described 6 patients who developed flattening of the cornea in the meridian that intersected a surgical or traumatic scar. He postulated that incisions of the cornea made at right angles to the steep meridian might be used to correct astigmatism.[10]

Lans,[11] a Dutch ophthalmologist, performed one of the first systematic studies of refractive surgery while at the University of Leiden in 1896. His doctoral thesis, titled *Experimental Studies of the Treatment of Astigmatism with Nonperforating Corneal Incisions*, described carefully planned experimentation in rabbits to evaluate patterns of keratotomy, keratectomy, and thermokeratoplasty. These studies also defined some basic principles of AK. Lans[11] showed that flattening in the meridian perpendicular to a transverse incision was associated with steepening in the opposite meridian and that the deeper and longer incisions had a greater effect.

Between 1940 and 1950,[12-15] Sato observed that spontaneous breaks in Descemet's membrane in patients with keratoconus could flatten the cornea and reduce their myopia. He and others in his group performed experiments on both posterior and anterior radial and AK incisions.[15-18] In addition, Sato discussed the concept of coupling, in which transverse incisions might be expected to flatten the steep meridian while simultaneously flattening the flatter meridian.[6] Sato, using a variety of techniques, used corneal incisions to reduce astigmatism.

In the 1970s, several surgeons in the Soviet Union studied myopic and astigmatic incisions.[19-23] In the mid-1970s, Fyodorov and Durnev[19,20] varied Sato's technique and introduced the concept of radial incisions performed only in the anterior peripheral cornea and sclera. Fyodorov and Durnev[23] devised a multifactorial formula using patient and surgical variables in an attempt to improve predictability of the procedure. Fyodorov and Durnev[19] then discussed using several anterior keratotomy patterns to correct myopic astigmatism. The use of RK to correct myopia and astigmatism in the United States was reported by Bores et al[24] in 1981. The National Eye Institute funded the Prospective Evaluation of Radial Keratotomy (PERK) study, which showed that unpredictability, refractive instability, and inadequate visual quality were still common with RK, despite improved techniques and refined nomograms.[25-30]

More recently, other investigators contributed to our understanding of AK results. The Astigmatism Reduction Clinical Trial (ARC-Trial), a prospective multicenter study published in 1995,[31] evaluated the predictability of the arcuate transverse keratotomy incisions using the Lindstrom nomogram. The ARC-Trial[31,32] evaluated patients with 1.00 to 6.00 D of corneal astigmatism and determined that the Lindstrom nomogram was an accurate guide for AK, with a tendency toward undercorrection. The ARC-Trial showed that the number and length of incisions, along with the age and the sex of the patient, determined the effectiveness of the incisions.[31,32] The Nichamin Age and Pachymetry-adjusted intralimbal arcuate Astigmatic (NAPA) nomogram is also widely used in ophthalmology currently.[32-35]

Since the advent of the femtosecond laser in the 1990s, it has been widely used in ophthalmology for creating corneal flaps in LASIK and in several steps of the cataract surgery itself. Recently, there has been interest in the use of the femtosecond laser for creating AK incisions at the time of cataract surgery. The femtosecond laser has already been used to create AK incision in patients following corneal grafts, and the results appear to be better than by using manual incision techniques.[35-43] The use of the femtosecond laser for creating LRIs is similar to the diamond blade for making incisions in the normal eye.[35,36,39,41-43] As such, this conversion may allow AK to continue to have a role at the time of IOL surgery for the correction of astigmatism. The femtosecond laser has the ability to cut at more precise depths and locations, which may result in more predictable corrections.

Currently, several systems are available or are in development. Although the LenSx (Alcon), LensAR (Lensar, Inc), OptiMedica (Abbott Medical Optics), Technolas Perfect Vision (Bausch & Lomb), and IntraLase (Abbott Medical Optics) all can create corneal incisions, the abilities of each system differ slightly, and some can also be used for anterior capsulotomy, lens fragmentation, and corneal incisions, such as relaxing incisions for astigmatism reduction.

The LenSx utilizes a disposable, curved interface that docks to the eye. It consists of an integrated ocular coherence tomography (OCT) imaging system that allows for real-time viewing of the anterior and posterior chambers. This technology makes it possible for surgeons to adjust cutting parameters before and during the procedure. The LenSx also has US Food and Drug Administration (FDA) approval for anterior capsulotomy and lens fragmentation procedures.[44,45]

The LensAR technology utilizes 3-dimensional, confocal-structured laser illumination, which is designed to improve depth of focus and improve imaging of more dense cataracts. This system is also portable. The LensAR currently has FDA approval for anterior capsulotomy and lens fragmentation procedures.[44,45]

OptiMedica combines a proprietary OCT with the Catalys Integral Guidance system, which allows for 3-dimensional mapping of the ocular structures. OptiMedica currently has FDA approval for anterior capsulotomy and lens fragmentation procedures.[44,45]

Technolas Perfect Vision uses real-time OCT, as well as a custom Curved Patient Interface with Intelligent Pressure sensors, which reduces corneal applanation.[44,45]

Abbott Medical Optics has the IntraLase femtosecond laser system, which is approved for femtosecond flap creation and keratoplasty incisions. As part of the keratoplasty incision software, relaxing incisions can be created.[46,47] A study has shown that these incisions can treat 0.25 to 2.50 D of astigmatism with high stability of the topography and refraction.[48] Work is ongoing in the development of software and hardware upgrades for incision and capsulorrhexis creation. Currently, Abbott Medical Optics has not received FDA approval for capsulorrhexis or lens fragmentation.

Toric IOLs are also able to reduce astigmatism at the time of cataract surgery. One study has compared the use of toric IOLs to manage more than 2.00 D of corneal astigmatism[48] with the results of peripheral corneal relaxing incisions.[49] The mean residual astigmatism after toric IOL implantation was 0.61 D compared with 1.32 D in those eyes with manual relaxing incisions. No difference in patient satisfaction was noted, yet a higher percentage of patients with relaxing incisions wore spectacles for distance correction. The amount of astigmatism, however, was higher than what is usually treated in the authors' practice (mean 1.82 ± 0.53 D). Typically, if the amount of correction is limited to <2.00 D, AK still works quite well. In addition, the presbyopic IOLs that are currently available in the United States do not incorporate toric versions, and the ease of AK and the increased use of the femtosecond laser make corneal relaxing incisions still a very attractive option for correcting astigmatism.

The Future

Despite continued competition between toric IOL implantation and AK, we anticipate a persistent role for corneal relaxing incisions. Because patients' expectations for uncorrected vision after cataract surgery continue to increase, the authors anticipate that attention to astigmatism correction will continue to grow, leading to a continued role for astigmatic incisions. In addition, continued growth in the lens-based refractive surgery field using the femtosecond laser will continue to make astigmatism incisions attractive, as they are able to be created by the femtosecond laser with more precision in placement and parameters, giving access to surgeons who have not previously felt comfortable with diamond blade–created incisions. Despite a current lack of data on the variability of response with the femtosecond laser, it is still anticipated that the depth, location, and precision of location may make a significant impact on managing corneal astigmatism in the foreseeable future.

During the preoperative planning for femtosecond laser relaxing incisions, the depth of the incisions posteriorly and anteriorly can be programmed, as well as the incisions' tilt from the anterior surface of the cornea. In addition, the optical zone anteriorly and posteriorly and the amount of stroma to remain anteriorly can be programmed into the laser. Thus, for the first time, one has the capability to perform intrastromal incisions, retaining an intact epithelium and Bowman's layer. This opens up additional options for creating the incisions that are still to be optimized through future studies. This also allows for the incisions to be further opened with a blunt tool later, if necessary.

The amount of effect that is obtained with incisions that are completely intrastromal is still being studied. Early reports suggest that approximately one-third to one-half the full amount can be obtained with anteriorly open incisions can be obtained with totally intrastromal incisions.

Table 1-1. Nomogram for Anterior Penetrating Relaxing Incisions With an 8.5-mm Optical Zone With the Femtosecond Laser

On-axis incision: 1.8 to 2.2 mm	0.25 D
On-axis incision: 2.8 to 3.2 mm	0.50 D
On-axis + 30 degrees CRI	0.75 D
On-axis + 45 degrees CRI	1.00 to 1.50 D
On-axis + 60 degrees CRI	1.50 to 2.00 D
2.25 D and higher	Toric IOL

Abbreviation: CRI, corneal relaxing incisions

Raoof-Daneshvar and Mian[49] suggested that multiple studies have demonstrated improved predictability and decreased complication rates when using the femtosecond laser to make the AK incisions.

The nomograms for using arcuate incisions with femtosecond lasers are not yet well tested; therefore, conservative nomograms are currently being used until the results are better known in an attempt to prevent overcorrection. The authors currently use this nomogram for anterior penetrating relaxing incisions with an 8.5-mm optical zone with the femtosecond laser (Table 1-1).

In the future, we will also see the increasing use of laser vision correction in patients after cataract surgery, even if AK was used at the time of initial surgery. These patients have significantly higher expectations for uncorrected vision after cataract surgery that the initial surgery does not always meet. If a patient does not reach his or her best visual potential and residual refractive error is to blame, he or she could use spectacles or contact lenses to manage residual refractive error. However, many patients desire reduced dependence on spectacles and contact lenses for daily activities. This will lead to increasing demand for postoperative laser vision correction such as photorefractive keratectomy (PRK).

Not all surgeons who perform lens surgery also perform laser vision correction. However, this does not mean that those surgeons cannot avail themselves of the benefits of laser vision correction after cataract surgery. In such cases, referral to a partner or colleague in the community who is a LASIK or PRK surgeon is often possible. A financial arrangement that makes sense for the laser refractive surgeon and the patient should be determined beforehand. However, most surgeons performing cataract surgery will benefit from the ability of performing laser vision correction also, as patient continuity typically increases patient satisfaction, and PRK is a learnable technique for cataract surgeons.

Conclusion

The principles of corneal relaxing incisions can be a useful adjunct in refining refractive outcomes at the time of small incision cataract surgery.[33,34,48,50] Because most surgeons prefer a single approach to most of their cases, the use of LRIs in conjunction with small incision cataract wound surgery is an effective method of astigmatism control.[33,34,48,50]

Various methods of incisional surgery have been utilized to correct astigmatism for many years. AK, to correct for corneal astigmatism, is less commonly performed as a primary procedure for the correction of refractive error, but it remains a useful adjunct at the time of cataract surgery, as visually significant astigmatism is common after cataract surgery.[33,34,50] There will be continued excitement about new technology such as toric IOLs and the use of femtosecond laser relaxing incisions at the time of cataract surgery; yet, LRIs in some format will continue to be utilized. Because of its accurate and successful ability to enhance refractive outcomes, laser vision enhancement will also be more frequently used. Careful testing of patients will still be important before the initial lens procedure, as well as for patients undergoing laser vision correction enhancements. Patient expectations and our ability to meet them will continue to grow.

References

1. Guyton DL. Prescribing cylinders the problem of distortions. *Surv Ophthalmol.* 1977;22(3):177-188.
2. Donders FC, Moore WD. *On the Anomalies of Accommodation and Refraction of the Eye: With a Preliminary Essay on Physiological Dioptrics.* London, England: New Sydenham Society; 1864.
3. Duke-Elder S, Stewart S, Abrams D. Ophthalmic optics and refraction. In: Duke-Elder S, ed. *System of Ophthalmology.* Vol 5. St Louis, MO: CV Mosby; 1970:274-295.
4. Chu R, Hardten R, Lindstrom R. Concepts in astigmatic keratotomy. In: Brightbill F, ed. *Corneal Surgery Theory, Techniques, and Tissue.* 3rd ed. St Louis, MO: Mosby; 1999:650-655.
5. Binder PS, Waring GO III. Keratotomy for astigmatism. In: Waring GO III, ed. *Refractive Keratotomy for Myopia and Astigmatism.* St Louis, MO: Mosby-Year Book; 1992:1085-1198.
6. Hardten DR, Lee S. Incisional keratotomy. In: Tasman W, ed. *Duane's Clinical Ophthalmology.* 2013 ed. Philadelphia, PA: Lippincott Williams & Wilkins; 2012:1-19.
7. Schiotz LJ. Hinfall von hochgradigem hornhautsastigmatismus nach staarextraction, besserung auf operativem wege. *Arch Augenheilkd.* 1885;15:178-181.
8. Faber E. Operative Behandeling van Astigmatisme. *Ned Tijdschr Geneeskd.* 1895;2:495-496.
9. Waring GO. History of radial keratotomy. In: Sanders D, Hofmann RD, Salz J, eds. *Refractive Corneal Surgery.* Thorofare, NJ: SLACK Incorporated; 1986:3-14.
10. Bates WH. A suggestion of an operation to correct astigmatism. *Arch Ophthalmol.* 1894;23:9-13.
11. Lans LJ. Experimentelle untersuchungen uber entstehung von astigmatismus durch nicperforirende corneawuden. *Graefes Arch Ophthalmol.* 1898;45:117-152.
12. Sato T. Treatment of conical cornea by incision of Descemet's membrane. *Acta Soc Ophthalmol Jpn.* 1939;43:541.
13. Sato T. Experimental study on surgical correction of astigmatism. *Juntendo Kenkyukaizasshi.* 1943;589:37-39.
14. Sato T. Posterior incision of the cornea: surgical treatment for conical cornea and astigmatism. *Am J Ophthalmol.* 1950;33)6):943-948.
15. Sato T. Die operative behandlung des astigmatismus. *Klin Monatsbl Augenheilkd.* 1955;126:16-31.
16. Akiyama K. Study of surgical treatment for myopia: II. Animal experimentation. *Acta Soc Ophthalmol Jpn.* 1955;59:294-312.
17. Sato T, Akiyama K, Shibata H. A new surgical approach to myopia. *Am J Ophthalmol.* 1953;36(61):823-829.
18. Akiyama K. The surgical treatment for myopia: III. Anterior and posterior incisions. *Acta Soc Ophthalmol Jpn.* 1955;59:797-853.
19. Fyodorov SN, Durnev VV. Surgical correction of complicated myopic astigmatism by means of dissection of circular ligament of cornea. *Ann Ophthalmol.* 1981;13(1):115-118.
20. Fyodorov SN, Durnev VV. Anterior keratotomy method application with the purpose of surgical correction of myopia. In: *Pressing Problems of Ophthalmosurgery.* Moscow, Russia: 1977:47-8.
21. Durnev VV. Decrease of corneal refraction by anterior keratotomy method with the purpose of surgical correction of myopia of mild to moderate degree. In: *Proceedings of the First Congress of Ophthalmologists of Transcaucasia, Tbilisi.* Moscow, Russia: Minister of Health, USSR; 1976:129-132.
22. Durnev VV, Ermoshin AS. Determination of dependence between length of anterior radial nonperforating incision of cornea and their effectiveness. In: *Transactions of the Fifth All-Union Conference of Inventors and Rationalizers in Ophthalmology Field.* Moscow, Russia: Minister of Health, USSR; 1976:106-108.
23. Fyodorov SN, Durnev VV. Operation of dosaged dissection of corneal circular ligament in cases of myopia of mild degree. *Ann Ophthalmol.* 1979;11(12):1885-1889.
24. Bores LD, Myers W, Cowden J. Radial keratotomy: an analysis of the American experience. *Ann Ophthalmol.* 1981;13(8):941-948.
25. Waring GO III, Moffitt SD, Gelender H, et al; the PERK Study Group. Rationale for and design of the National Eye Institute Prospective Evaluation of Radial Keratotomy (PERK) Study. *Ophthalmology.* 1983;90(1):40-58.
26. Waring GO, Lynn MJ, Fielding B, et al. Results of the Prospective Evaluation of Radial Keratotomy (PERK) study 4 years after surgery for myopia. Perk Study Group. *JAMA.* 1990;263(8):1083-1091.

27. Waring GO III, Lynn MJ, Nizam A, et al. Results of the Prospective Evaluation of Radial Keratotomy (PERK) Study five years after surgery. *Ophthalmology.* 1991;98(8):1164-1176.
28. Bullock JD, Lindquist TD, eds. Radial keratotomy for myopia: Committee on Ophthalmic Procedures Assessment approved by Board of Directors, American Academy of Ophthalmology. *Ophthalmology.* 1993;100:1113.
29. Waring GO III, Lynn MJ, McDonnell PJ. Results of the Prospective Evaluation of Radial Keratotomy (PERK) study 10 years after surgery. *Arch Ophthalmol.* 1994;112(10):1298-1308.
30. Leaming DV. Practice styles and preferences of ASCRS members—1999 survey. *J Cataract Refract Surg.* 2000;26(6):913-921.
31. Price FW, Grene RB, Marks RG, Gonzales JS. Astigmatism reduction clinical trial: a multicenter prospective evaluation of the predictability of arcuate keratotomy. Evaluation of surgical nomogram predictability. ARC-T Study Group. *Arch Ophthalmol.* 1995;113(3):277-282.
32. Nichamin LD. Astigmatism control. *Ophthalmol Clin North Am.* 2006;19(4):485-493.
33. Nichamin LD. Treating astigmatism at the time of cataract surgery. *Curr Opin Ophthalmol.* 2003;14(1):35-38.
34. Nichamin LD. Astigmatism management for modern phaco surgery. *Int Ophthalmol Clin.* 2003;43(3):53-63.
35. Harissi-Dagher M, Azar DT. Femtosecond laser astigmatic keratotomy for postkeratoplasty astigmatism. *Can J Ophthalmol.* 2008;43(3):367-369.
36. Buzzonetti L, Petrocelli G, Laborante A, Mazzilli E, Gaspari M, Valente P. Arcuate keratotomy for high postoperative keratoplasty astigmatism performed with the Intralase femtosecond laser. *J Refract Surg.* 2009;25(8):709-714.
37. Hoffart L, Proust H, Matonti F, Conrath J, Ridings B. Correction of postkeratoplasty astigmatism by femtosecond laser compared with mechanized astigmatic keratotomy. *Am J Ophthalmol.* 2009;147(5):779-787.
38. Kymionis GD, Yoo SH, Ide T, Culbertson WW. Femtosecond-assisted astigmatic keratotomy for post-keratoplasty irregular astigmatism. *J Cataract Refract Surg.* 2009;35(1):11-13.
39. Nubile M, Carpineto P, Lanzini M, et al. Femtosecond laser arcuate keratotomy for the correction of high astigmatism after keratoplasty. *Ophthalmology.* 2009;116(6):1083-1092.
40. Yoo SH, Kymionis GD, Ide T, Diakonis VF. Overcorrection after femtosecond-assisted astigmatic keratotomy in a post-Descemet-stripping automated endothelial keratoplasty patient. *J Cataract Refract Surg.* 2009;35(10):1833-1834.
41. Kumar NL, Kaiserman I, Shehadeh-Mashor R, Sansanayudh W, Ritenour R, Rootman DS. IntraLase-enabled astigmatic keratotomy for post-keratoplasty astigmatism:on-axis vector analysis. *Ophthalmology.* 2010;117(6):1228-1235.
42. Vaddavalli PK, Humeric V, Yoo SH. Air bubble in anterior chamber as indicator of full-thickness incisions in femtosecond-assisted astigmatic keratotomy. *J Cataract Refract Surg.* 2011;37(9):1723-1725.
43. Wu E. Femtosecond-assisted astigmatic keratotomy. *Int Ophthalmol Clin.* 2011;51(2):77-85.
44. Uy HS, Edwards K, Curtis N. Femtosecond phacoemulsification: the business and the medicine. *Curr Opin Ophthalmol.* 2012;23(2):33-39.
45. Larkin H. Femtosecond lasers: four systems are on the market or close to launch. *Eurotimes.* 2011;16:10.
46. Rueckl T, Dexl AK, Reischl V, Binder PS, Bor Z, Grabner G. Intrastromal arcuate keratotomy using a femtosecond laser. Paper presented at: American Academy of Ophthalmology 2011 Annual Meeting; October 22-25, 2011; Orlando, FL.
47. Mamalis N. Correction of astigmatism during cataract surgery. *J Cataract Refract Surg.* 2009;35(3):403-404.
48. Mingo-Botín D, Muñoz-Negrete FJ, Won Kim HR, Morcillo-Laiz R, Rebolleda G, Oblanca N. Comparison of toric intraocular lenses and peripheral corneal relaxing incisions to treat astigmatism during cataract surgery. *J Cataract Refract Surg.* 2010;36(10):1700-1708.
49. Raoof-Daneshvar D, Mian SI. Femtosecond laser-assisted astigmatism correction. In: Goggin M, ed. *Astigmatism—Optics, Physiology, and Management.* Rijeka, Croatia: InTech; 2012.
50. Gills JP. Treating astigmatism at the time of cataract surgery. *Curr Opin Ophthalmol.* 2002;13(1):2-6.

2

Measuring Astigmatism
Planning Surgery and Tracking Results

Noel A. Alpins, MD, FACS and George Stamatelatos, OD

Measuring Astigmatism

Limbal relaxing incisions (LRIs) are used to change the shape of the cornea and reduce astigmatism both on the cornea and in the resulting refractive cylinder. Numerous clinical devices are available to determine corneal and refractive astigmatism values. Both modes of measurement—corneal and refractive—may be assessed and considered when determining the amount of astigmatism that needs to be reduced and at which meridian to place the LRIs.

Topography Systems

Corneal topography, which uses computer-assisted video keratography (CAVK), measures and calculates 8000 to 10,000 points on the anterior corneal surface to determine elevation and power. Many topographers also measure the posterior corneal surface. This permits the determination of regional corneal thickness, as well as the posterior corneal shape, so that irregular conditions and ectasias can be detected. The simulated keratometry (Sim K) gauge of astigmatism is calculated using the central 3-mm region of the cornea. This parameter was introduced in the 1980s to parallel manual keratometry readings. The more recent description of corneal topographic astigmatism now provides a more accurate means to quantify corneal astigmatism.[1]

Corneal topography is an essential component to the work-up and assessment of the astigmatic surgical candidate for both the measurement of cylinder and for the detection of subtle pathology, such as keratoconus or pellucid marginal degeneration; conditions that might preclude the use of incisional surgery, such as LRI procedures.

Manual Keratometry

Corneal curvature using traditional manual keratometry entails measurement at only 4 points within 3 to 4 mm of the central anterior corneal surface. Distortion of the keratometry mires indicates corneal irregularity—the greater the distortion of the mires, the greater the corneal unevenness.

Nichamin LD.
Limbal Relaxing Incisions: A Practical Guide (pp 15-25).

Manifest Refraction

The manifest refractive cylinder represents a subjective means of measurement. It incorporates perceptual astigmatism, as well as whole eye astigmatism. In many cases, the refractive cylinder will be different in magnitude and/or orientation to the corneal astigmatism; however, in the case of planning LRIs, the surgeon may want to base the surgical parameters on a combination of both. The manifest refractive cylinder is usually expressed in steps of 0.25 diopters (D).

Wavefront Refraction

Wavefront (aberrometry) refraction is an ocular measurement of astigmatism, independent of subjective and central neural processing. Although the second-order spherocylinder can be measured in 0.01-D steps, utilizing this modality, compared with 0.25-D steps in manifest refraction, must correlate closely with the manifest refraction for both spherical and astigmatic components before its accuracy can be confirmed.

To achieve high accuracy with wavefront measurements, it is important to avoid excess accommodation. To this end, the patient should avoid near work for approximately 15 minutes before a measurement is taken, and it is preferable to spend this period of time in a darkened room to promote pupillary dilation, thereby maximizing the detection of higher-order aberrations.

Regardless of which measurement is adopted for clinical use, it is recommended that the same instrument be used to measure both the preoperative and the postoperative parameters for analysis. Ideally, it is also recommended that the same clinician or technician perform these measurements.

Planning Surgery

The planning of LRI procedures performed at the time of cataract surgery is best based on and more highly weighted toward corneal parameters. Measures of manifest or wavefront refractive astigmatism may not be accurate due to the coexisting cataract, and subsequent removal of the natural crystalline lens of the eye will impact the final refractive outcome. Furthermore, the amount of corneal astigmatism requiring correction and its orientation must take into account the induced effect of the phaco incision. This can most accurately be determined by analyzing previous phaco incisions of the same size and calculating a mean flattening effect at the appropriate corneal meridia around the eye (Figure 2-1).

Different techniques can be applied when LRIs are used to correct corneal astigmatism:

1. **Using the Phaco Incision as One of the Pair of LRIs.** With this method, the position of the phaco incision will vary, depending on the steep meridian of the preoperative corneal astigmatism. The phaco incision needs to "mimic" the effect of the opposing LRI. Therefore, it will need to be made wider and, in some cases, be positioned slightly more centrally to gain a more pronounced flattening effect than typically induced when phaco incisions are used solely to remove the natural lens or to insert an intraocular lens (IOL).

   The LRI will then be placed 180 degrees away from this phaco incision. It is recommended that the LRI be performed prior to the phaco incision, as the eye is firmer at this stage, thereby allowing for a more accurate length and depth of the LRI.

   With this technique, there is no need to allow for any "off-axis" effects[2] due to the phaco incision—the phaco incision is positioned precisely on the steep corneal meridian.

   The theoretical reduction effect is calculated arithmetically when placed at the steep meridian (Figure 2-2). This technique requires 2 incisions in total.

2. **Using a Phaco Incision Together With Paired LRIs.** Placing a phaco incision away from the steepest corneal meridian will have an "off-axis" rotational effect on the preoperative corneal

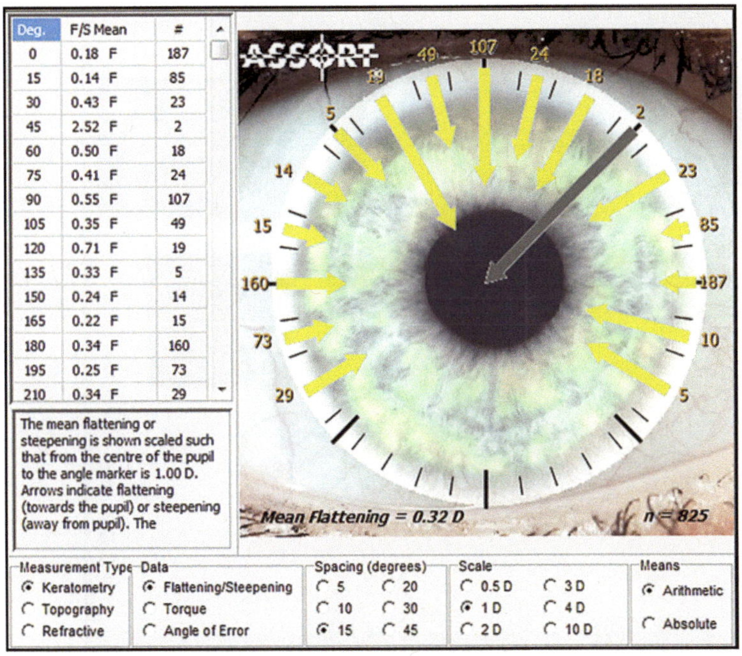

Figure 2-1. Display of the flattening effect by keratometry of 2.2-mm phaco incisions for both the left and right eyes where the incision is placed at the steepest corneal meridian. The varying sizes of the arrows indicate the varying amounts of flattening—the longer the arrow, the greater the flattening.

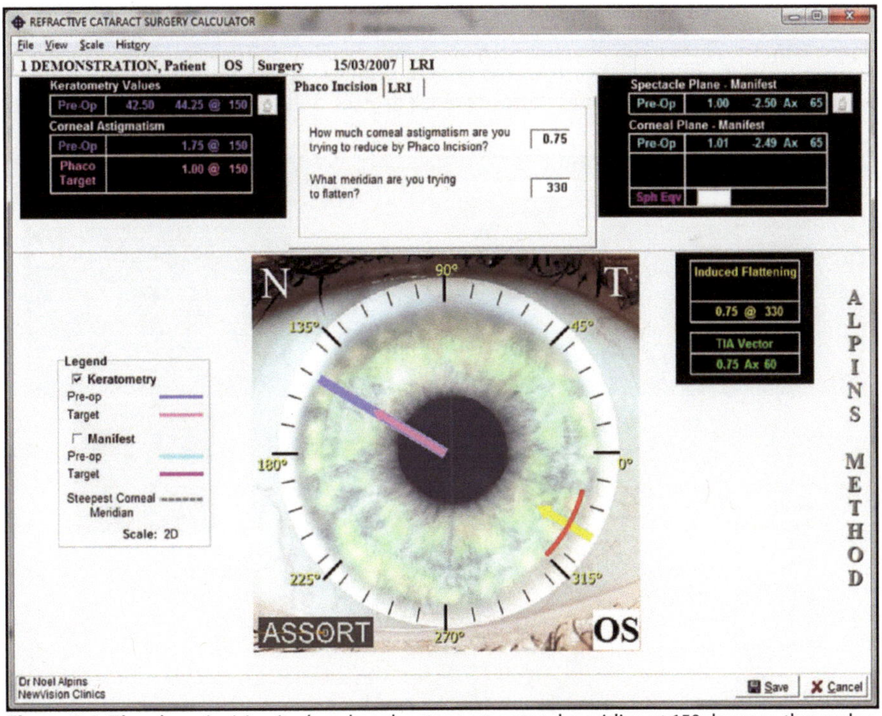

Figure 2-2. The phaco incision is placed on the steepest corneal meridian at 150 degrees, thus reducing the corneal astigmatism from the preoperative amount of 1.75 to 1.00 D. The red line indicates phaco incision and the yellow line is the amount of associated flattening. Abbreviation: N, nasal; T, temporal.

astigmatism (Figure 2-3A). This must be taken into account when planning for the effect required from the additional pair of LRIs and their positioning (Figure 2-3B). This technique requires a total of 3 incisions.

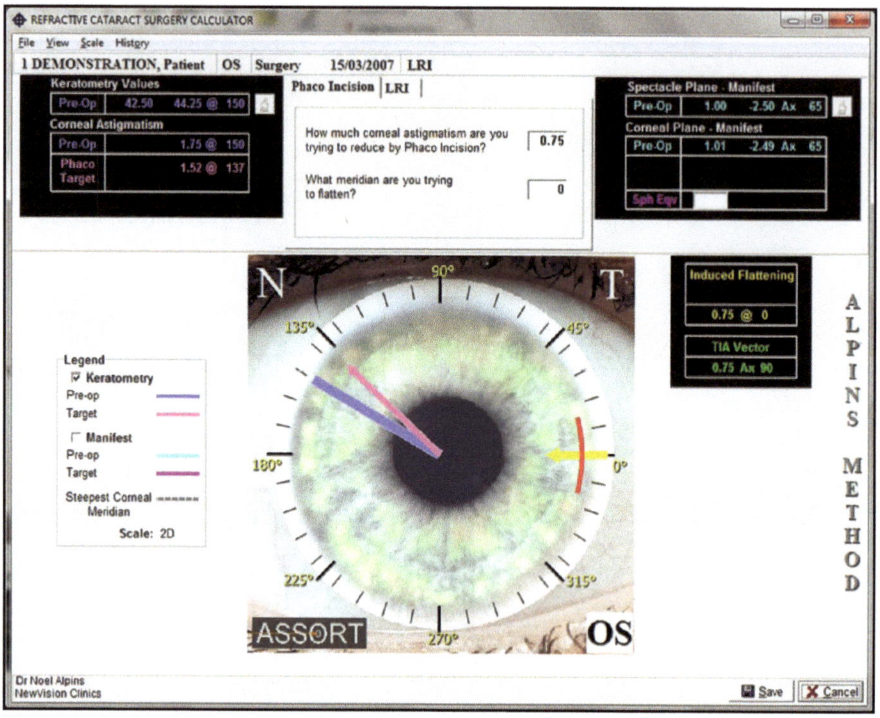

Figure 2-3A. The phaco incision is placed temporally at a meridian of 0 degrees, reducing the preoperative corneal astigmatism of 1.75 to 1.52 D. Note that the steepest corneal meridian has now rotated 13 degrees from 150 degrees clockwise to 137 degrees. Abbreviations: N, nasal; T, temporal.

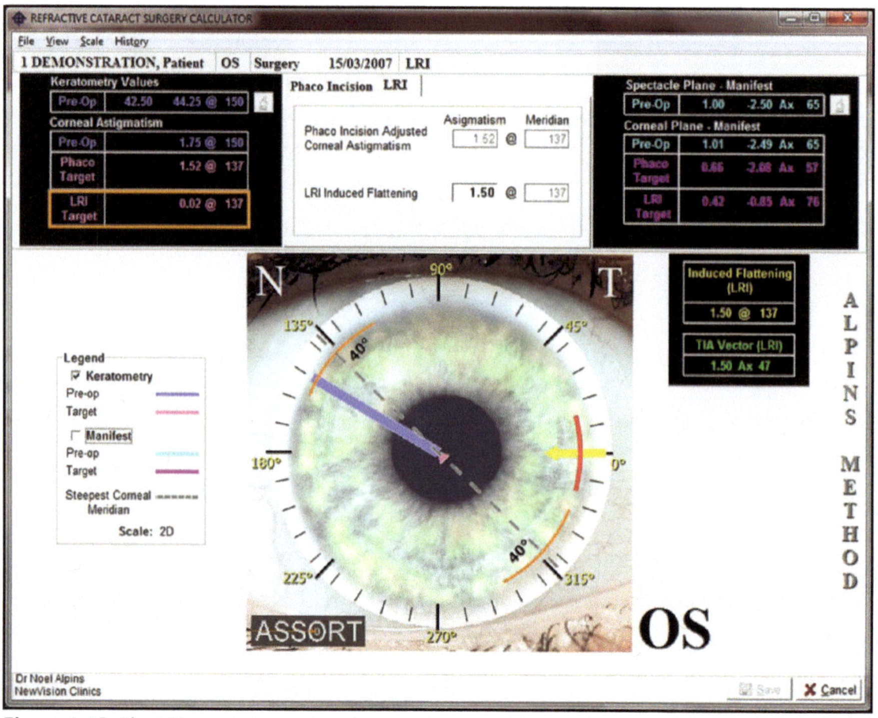

Figure 2-3B. The LRI incisions are placed at the steep meridian of the (phaco) incision-adjusted corneal astigmatism at 137 degrees, instead of the preoperative steep meridian of 150 degrees. The red line indicates phaco incision, the yellow line is the amount of associated flattening, and the orange lines indicate the LRI incisions. Abbreviations: N, nasal; T, temporal.

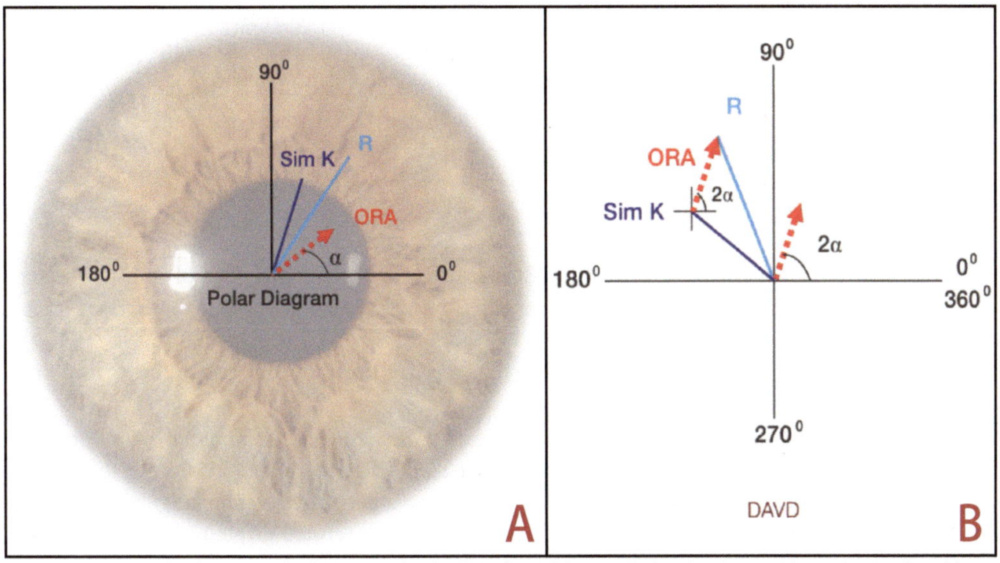

Figure 2-4. (A) Polar diagram of refractive cylinder (R in figure) (corneal plane) at its positive axis, simulated keratometry steep meridian and ORA as they would appear on the eye. (B) Double-angle vector diagram (DAVD) showing a "doubling" of both the positive cylinder axes without a change in the astigmatic magnitudes.

3. **Paired LRIs Not Associated With a Phaco Incision.** If the natural lens of the eye is clear and will not be removed and if correction of the total astigmatism of the eye is required, then both the corneal and refractive astigmatism (corneal plane) can be considered when planning the effect of the LRIs; the most effective magnitude and position of the LRI will lie somewhere between the 2 corneal and refractive astigmatisms. Using this optimization method, it is important to calculate ocular residual astigmatism (ORA) preoperatively. The ORA is the vectorial difference between the corneal astigmatism and the refractive cylinder at the corneal plane and is expressed in diopters (Figure 2-4).[3,4] The greater the ORA, the more astigmatism will be left uncorrected postoperatively in the optical system of the eye, regardless of how precisely the procedure was performed. A routine assessment of the ORA preoperatively allows the surgeon to advise the patient accordingly on the expected visual outcome. If the ORA is high (>1.00 D), depending on the amount of preoperative astigmatism, the visual outcome may not meet the patient's expectations. Therefore, the patient should be advised accordingly prior to surgery so that he or she is able to achieve realistic expectations regarding the likely outcome of surgery.

Limbal Relaxing Incision Nomograms

A number of nomograms currently exist that determine the length of the LRIs:

1. *The NAPA (Nichamin Age and Pachymetry-Adjusted) Nomogram* (Dr. Louis D. "Skip" Nichamin) in which the length of the incision decreases with age and increases with the magnitude of astigmatism requiring correction.
2. *The DONO Nomogram* (Dr. Eric D. Donnenfeld) in which the length of the incision increases with increasing magnitude of astigmatism correction.
3. *The Gills LRI Nomogram* (Dr. James P. Gills) titrates surgery by the length and number of LRIs.

4. *The Wallace LRI Nomogram* (Dr. R. Bruce Wallace III) in which the number of LRIs and their length increases as the amount of astigmatism correction increases and decreases with age.

Many other surgeons, such as Drs. Thornton, Lindstrom, and Buzzard, have their own variation of one of these commonly used nomograms or have developed their own personal LRI nomograms determined from retrospective analyses of their own data.

Tracking Results

To analyze LRI astigmatic outcomes, the postoperative corneal astigmatism of an individual eye must be compared with its preoperative corneal astigmatism vectorially. The astigmatic treatment intended by the LRIs must be known, recorded, and compared with the vectorial result—the surgically induced astigmatism vector (SIA), which is the vectorial difference between the postoperative and preoperative corneal astigmatism.

The target-induced astigmatism vector (TIA) is the amount of astigmatism the surgeon is attempting to correct, using either paired LRIs or the TIA from the phaco incision (if this is being used as one of the LRIs) plus the TIA from the opposing LRI, added vectorially. The difference vector is the correction that would be required to achieve the intended target of the initial surgery. If the initial surgery is successful, then the difference vector is zero.

The various relationships between these 3 vectors form the basis of the Alpins method and allow for a basic analysis that determines whether the astigmatism was overcorrected or undercorrected and whether the treatment was on- or off-axis.[5-7]

Correction Index

The correction index (CI) is the amount of astigmatism correction achieved. It is calculated by dividing the SIA by the TIA; the ideal value is 1.0. Correction index values greater than 1.0 indicate an overcorrection, and values less than 1.0 indicate an undercorrection.

Angle of Error

The angle of error (AE) is the angle between the TIA and the SIA on a polar diagram. The AE is positive if the SIA is counterclockwise to the TIA, and it is negative if the SIA is clockwise to the TIA.

Magnitude of Error

The magnitude of error (ME) is the arithmetic difference between the magnitudes of the SIA and the TIA. ME is positive for an overcorrection and negative for an undercorrection.

Index of Success

The index of success (IOS) is calculated by dividing the difference vector by the TIA. The IOS is a relative measure of success. It takes into account the targeted amount of astigmatism correction preoperatively. Ideally, when the target is achieved at the first application of a corrective procedure, the IOS is zero.

Coefficient of Adjustment

The coefficient of adjustment (CA) is the factor required to adjust future astigmatism treatment magnitudes and is calculated by dividing the TIA by the SIA. Ideally, the value is 1.0; it is the inverse of the CI. The CA of 1.0 is the nomogram adjustment that is applied to either the angular length of the arcuate incisions or to the position (optical zone) of the arcuate incisions relative to the center of the cornea.

Flattening Effect

The flattening effect (FE) of the phaco incision must be calculated over time to improve accuracy. This is done by using a double-angle vector diagram (DAVD), where the effect of the SIA on

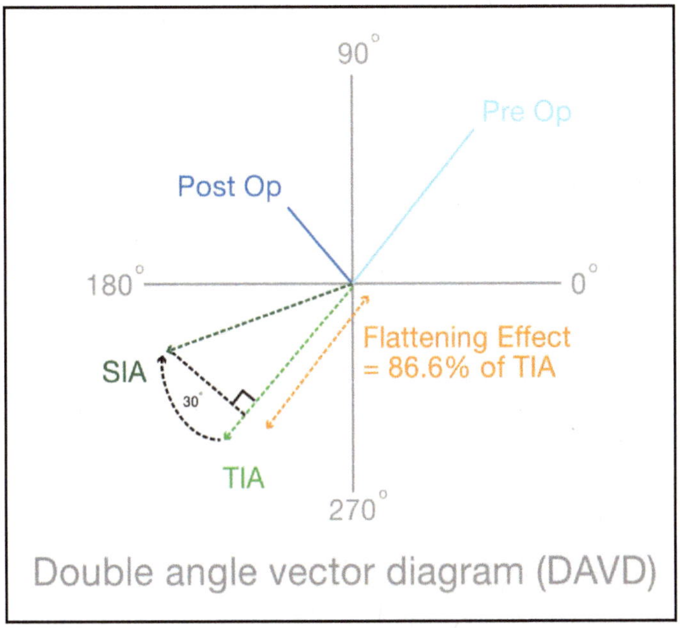

Figure 2-5. The FE demonstrates the effect of the SIA at the intended astigmatic treatment meridian when misaligned by 15 degrees and is expressed in diopters with a loss of effect of 13.4%.

the TIA axis is calculated using trigonometric principles (Figure 2-5). The DAVD is then converted to a polar diagram to display how the FE would appear on an eye. The average flattening for any particular meridian can then be used for future phaco procedures to determine the expected effect on the preoperative corneal astigmatism at that position on the cornea.

The FE is defined as: FE = SIA cos 2.AE[2,6]

Individual Outcomes

A single LRI procedure can be analyzed using vector analysis; however, no nomogram adjustment can be performed without aggregating data from multiple eyes. A one-by-one case analysis can determine the magnitude of the additional astigmatic treatment required and can determine at what meridian any further surgical enhancement should occur, as well as the relative success indicators of any one procedure.

Astigmatism Sign Convention

To assist with the following examples, it is useful to be aware of sign convention as it applies to astigmatism and vectors.

The convention sign "@" refers to the steep corneal meridian and the greatest power. The "Ax" or "x," representing the axis notation, refers to a position 90 degrees away from the steep corneal meridian, which is zero or the least refractive power of a cylindrical lens, such as the negative cylinder axis in a manifest refraction. Vectors, which must always be positive, are aligned with this negative cylinder axis, so their notation is always "Ax" and never "@." An incision that flattens the steep meridian and an ablation that steepens the flat meridian 90 degrees away will share the same TIA (treatment vector) axis because they are having the same net astigmatic effect.

For example, we assume a scenario where the preoperative corneal astigmatism has been measured as 2.50 D Ax 68 (minus cylinder) in the left eye, and the LRI procedure has been planned to correct 2.00 D of this astigmatism. The analysis is based on a resultant target of 0.50 D corneal astigmatism as the aim of this corrective procedure.

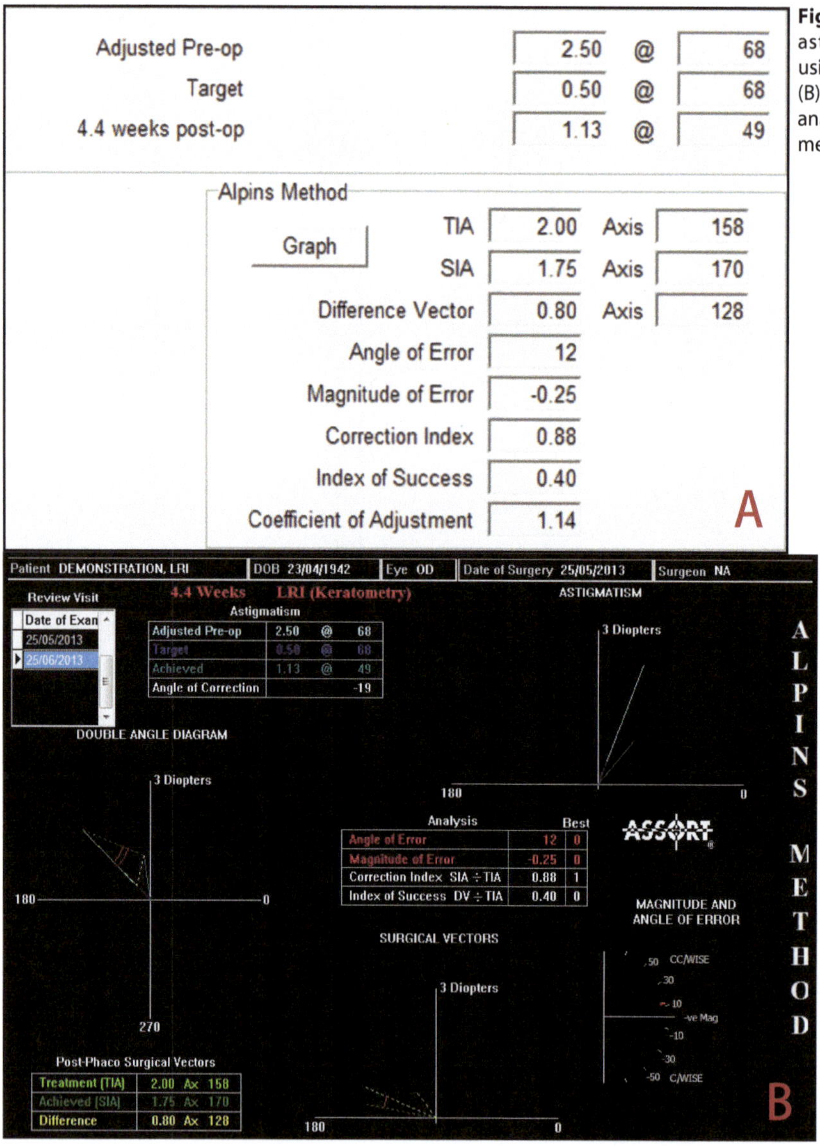

Figure 2-6. (A) Numerical astigmatism analysis using the Alpins method. (B) Graphical astigmatism analysis using the Alpins method.

The achieved (postoperative) corneal astigmatism is measured at 1.13 D @ 49.

Figure 2-6A displays the numerical astigmatism analysis and Figure 2-6B shows the graphical astigmatism analysis, using the Alpins method for the previous example.

The TIA is 2.00 D, which is the planned correction of the LRIs. It is at an axis of 158 degrees, that is, 90 degrees away from the planned meridian to be flattened, as vectors create a steepening change.

The SIA was calculated to be 1.75 D Ax 170.

Did the LRI Procedure Over- or Undercorrect the Astigmatism?

This is determined by calculating the CI as CI = SIA/TIA = 1.75/2.00 D = 0.88. The astigmatism was therefore undercorrected by 12%.

Were the LRIs On- or Off-Axis?

This can be determined by using the AE between the TIA and the SIA. In the previous example, it is 12 degrees counterclockwise. The LRIs were planned to be at 68 degrees, but postoperative analysis determine that they were in fact functionally placed at 80 degrees.

The FE of this LRI procedure is 1.61 D Ax 158, which is less than the intended effect of 2.00 D (TIA). It is also less than the SIA, as it is off-axis by 12 degrees, causing loss of effect.

Aggregate Outcomes

Aggregate Analysis Data

When adjusting nomograms, it is important to have at least 50 cases, with 3-month postoperative data that can be analyzed. This is to ensure that any trends observed are statistically valid and consistent, and the effect of isolated outliers is minimized. Two types of analysis are relevant:

1. Arithmetic means: astigmatism vector magnitudes are averaged, irrespective of their orientation.
2. Summated vector means (SVM): head-to-tail summation of vectors.

Systematic errors can be gauged by comparing the SVM and the arithmetic mean magnitudes. The greater the difference between the arithmetic and the SVM's magnitudes, the more likely it is that the changes occurring are a result of random events. A ratio above 0.6 and close to 1.0 indicates that the trend achieved by the surgery is consistent and predictable.

Non-Zero Targets

When analyzing outcomes of LRIs, one must consider the difference between preoperative corneal astigmatism and the amount of astigmatism the procedure is able to correct. Note that it is the intended corneal astigmatism that the procedure will correct, so if the nomogram used indicates that only 1.50 D and not 2.00 D of astigmatism can be corrected by using a particular degree of arc, the analysis should be based on a non-zero astigmatic target of 0.50 D. The nomogram is calculated on the amount of astigmatism intended and not on what might have been unrealistically desired.

Misalignment of Limbal Relaxing Incisions

If an LRI is misaligned with the intended meridian, the cause for the loss of astigmatic effect may be misleading when calculated vectorially. A misalignment of 15 degrees will actually result in a 13.4% loss in the astigmatic effect of the treatment; a 30-degree misalignment will result in a loss in astigmatic effect of 50%.[2] This can be demonstrated by postoperatively measuring the astigmatism at the same intended preoperative treatment meridian and NOT at the postoperative steep meridian. This measurement is acquired by using a keratometer and comparing this *measured value* to the preoperative astigmatism at its meridian (Figure 2-7). Note that this is a magnitude-only comparison. Complete loss of effect occurs at 45 degrees off axis. At this position, the SIA, which is still prevailing, is acting wholly as torque; it rotates the astigmatism rather than reducing it.

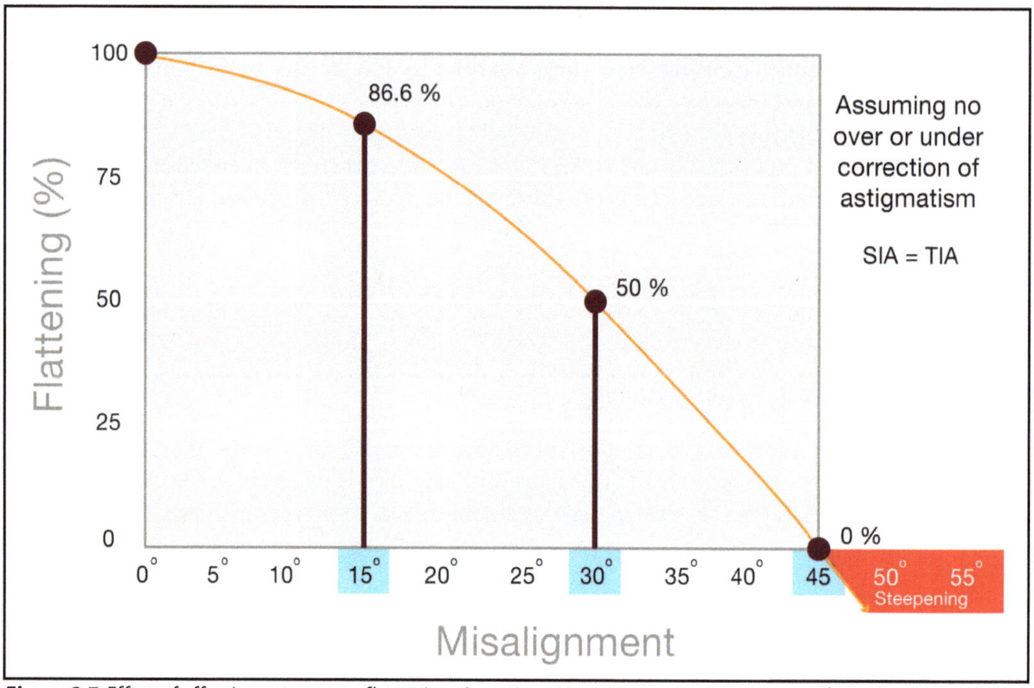

Figure 2-7. Effect of off-axis treatment on flattening. An astigmatic treatment 30 degrees away from the *intended* treatment meridian will result in a 50% loss in flattening at the intended meridian.

Conclusion

Astigmatism can be measured by using both corneal and refractive modalities—consistency of both equipment and operator is the key to accuracy, but in practice, these commonly differ, contributing in part to our inability to completely eliminate astigmatism.

Planning LRI procedures should incorporate all available astigmatism measurements together with surgeon-specific outcome data to help predict the effect of the phaco and/or the LRI incisions. An understanding of the vectorial changes that occur will assist in the refinement and optimal application of nomograms. Regular postoperative astigmatic analyses of LRI procedures allow for ongoing nomogram refinement and hence potential for continual improvement in visual outcomes of future surgery.

References

1. Alpins NA, Ong JK, Stamatelatos G. New method of quantifying corneal topographic astigmatism that corresponds with manifest refractive cylinder. *J Cataract Refract Surg.* 2012;38(11):1978-1988.
2. Alpins NA. Vector analysis of astigmatism changes by flattening, steepening, and torque. *J Cataract Refract Surg.* 1997;23(10):1503-1514.
3. Alpins NA. New method of targeting vectors to treat astigmatism. *J Cataract Refract Surg.* 1997;23(1):65-75.
4. Kugler L, Cohen I. Haddad W, Wang MX. Efficacy of laser in situ keratomileusis in correcting anterior and non-anterior corneal astigmatism: comparative study. *J Cataract Refract Surg.* 2010;36(10):1745-1752.

5. Alpins NA. A new method of analyzing vectors for changes in astigmatism. *J Cataract Refract Surg.* 1993;19(4):524-533.
6. Alpins NA. Astigmatism analysis by the Alpins method. *J Cataract Refract Surg.* 2001;27(1):31-49.
7. Wikipedia contributors. Alpins method of astigmatism analysis. *Wikipedia, The Free Encyclopedia.* October 19, 2013, 13:56 UTC. http://en.wikipedia.org/w/index.php?title=Alpins_method_of_astigmatism_analysis&oldid=577844863. Accessed June 6, 2012,

3

Overview for the Use of Limbal Relaxing Incisions

Louis D. "Skip" Nichamin, MD

When assessing the recent changes in modern cataract and intraocular lens (IOL) implantation surgery, arguably, the single most pressing challenge facing today's phacoemulsification (phaco) surgeon is the need to achieve predictable and accurate refractive outcomes. Similarly, one might view the most common complication of contemporary IOL surgery to be the persistence of residual and symptomatic refractive error. Indeed, the fields of cataract and refractive surgery have all but merged to form a single amalgam, and surgeons and patients alike have come to largely measure the success of their surgery by the refractive outcome. Furthermore, one of the leading causes for litigation in our field is the "refractive surprise."[1] As mentioned in the Introduction, the refractive lens exchange has now become an important component of the refractive surgeon's armamentarium and, in many cases, the preferred technique for presbyopic patients.[2] Improved refractive results in lens-based surgery have come about by way of advances in both surgical technique and innovative changes in technology. For example, spherical results have become more predictable because of increased attention to biometry techniques, as well as breakthrough technology such as partial coherence interferometry.[3]

Just as important is the astigmatic component of the refractive equation. At one time during the evolution of small-incision surgery, it was the surgeon's goal to simply not induce astigmatism.[4] Today, to fully embrace the concept of "refractive cataract surgery," one must be able to assess, reduce, and in some cases, eliminate pre-existing cylinder.

Patient Selection and Considerations

Estimates of the incidence of significant, naturally occurring astigmatism vary widely, ranging from 7.5% to 75%.[5] It has been reported that 3% to 15% of eyes may have 2 or more diopters (D) of astigmatism.[6] In the author's clinical experience, 10% of patients presenting for surgery have >2.00 D, 20% have between 1.00 and 2.00 D, and 70% have <1.00 D of pre-existing cylinder. In light of the recent experience gained in the field of keratorefractive surgery, most surgeons would agree that astigmatism >0.50 D will lead to symptoms of ghosting and shadows. Although the older cataract patient may be more tolerant of cylinder, the ambitious refractive cataract surgeon should approach a patient for implant with the same high goals that he or she might with a younger keratorefractive candidate, aiming for both a spherical and astigmatic outcome of ±0.50 D.[7] As

Nichamin LD.
Limbal Relaxing Incisions: A Practical Guide (pp 27-46).

such, approximately 35% of patients requiring implant surgery will likely need some form of astigmatism correction to achieve reasonable, unaided visual function.

When considering astigmatism surgery, one must take into account the location of the cylinder, the age of the patient, and the status of the fellow eye. Because most patients will drift against-the-rule (ATR) over their lifetime—for example, toward plus cylinder at 180 degrees—some surgeons have advocated a less aggressive approach to the reduction of with-the-rule (WTR) cylinder. Other authors have also suggested that residual WTR astigmatism may favor better uncorrected distance acuity, given that most visual stimuli are of a vertical nature.[8] Similarly, it has been contended that ATR cylinder may improve uncorrected near vision.[9] Furthermore, some have held to the tenet that residual (myopic) WTR astigmatism is a desirable goal to enlarge the conoid of Sturm and hence optimize depth perception. Such theories that contend that residual refractive error may, in some way, be beneficial to the patient have more recently been called into question.[10,11] With recent refinements in surgical technique that permit more precise outcomes, along with increased performance demands required for presbyopia-correcting IOLs, a spherical result has become the goal for the majority of patients undergoing implant surgery.

Treatment Options

The first decision faced by the surgeon is whether to address pre-existing astigmatism at the time of cataract and IOL surgery or to defer and treat the cylinder separately. One could reasonably argue that for optimal accuracy, sufficient time for wound healing should be allotted, and a stable refraction ought to be documented prior to astigmatic correction. This consideration may have been more germane with the use of earlier and previously larger incisions, but with modern foldable IOLs and injector delivery devices that now routinely permit wound sizes of 2.5 mm or less, many studies have documented the nearly neutral astigmatic effect that these incisions bear, as well as their early refractive stability.[12-14] As such, most surgeons feel that concomitant treatment of pre-existing astigmatism is a more efficient approach, and it is favored because it will likely save the patient from having to undergo a second procedure.

The next major decision is whether to treat the astigmatism through a lenticular approach; that is, to use a toric IOL or to utilize a keratorefractive technique. From a theoretical perspective, it is hard to argue against the use of toric implants, and their effectiveness has been widely reported.[15] This approach has the potential to avoid induced irregular astigmatism from corneal manipulation and provides the option of reversibility. In the United States, only 2 toric IOL offerings exist, and, at the time of this printing, no premium presbyopic-correcting implant has been approved by the US Food and Drug Administration. Even with the availability of toric lenses, limbal relaxing incisions (LRIs) serve a useful role as an enhancement technique following use of these implants and expand the IOL's range of correction. LRIs are also frequently used in conjunction with phakic IOLs and may improve excimer laser results by decreasing cylindric ablation zones and permit wider ranges of astigmatic correction.[16]

The notion of reducing astigmatism at the time of cataract surgery by way of astigmatic keratotomy was first proposed by Robert Osher and dates back to the mid-1980s.[17-19] The author's personal experience with this technique began in 1988 and was based on the principles of astigmatic keratotomy, as taught by Dr. Spencer Thornton.[20] A transition to (intra) LRIs took place in 1994, which was spurred by the experience of Dr. Dave Dillman and his improved results using the peripheral limbal technique of Dr. Stephen Hollis, who was an early advocate and innovator in the use of LRIs (oral communication). With refinement of the Hollis nomogram, we found this more peripheral approach to astigmatic keratotomy to be considerably more forgiving than conventional astigmatic keratotomy performed at a smaller (ie, 7.0 mm) optical zone.[21-23]

Before delving into more detail regarding the use of LRIs, other approaches to address pre-existing cylinder should be noted. For example, one can, to a limited degree, decrease nominal amounts of astigmatism by manipulating the main phaco and implant incision. By first placing the incision on the steep corneal meridian and then by varying its size and design, one can affect a desired amount of wound flattening, and hence a decrease in cylinder.[24] Specifically, one can increase or decrease the amount of wound flattening by increasing or decreasing the size of the incision. Similarly, wound flattening may be enhanced by moving closer to the visual axis or by creating a more circum-parallel incision to the limbus (as opposed to a more neutral "frown" configuration). Also, a perpendicular component (or groove) may be added to the incision to further increase wound flattening and "against-the-wound" astigmatic drift.[20] However, such an approach presents logistical challenges, including movement around the surgical table, which often produces awkward hand positions. In addition, varying surgical instrumentation may be needed, along with a dynamic mindset, and this approach is effective only for relatively small degrees of pre-existing cylinder. For these reasons, this technique has largely been supplanted by the use of a consistent and essentially neutral phaco incision, typically located temporally for astigmatic stability, and then adding supplemental relaxing incisions (LRIs). A study by Kaufmann et al[25] concluded that LRIs in combination with a temporal clear corneal incision provided superior astigmatic outcomes compared with "on-axis" (a misnomer, as discussed in Chapter 2) surgery.[25]

Another novel incisional approach—the use of opposing clear corneal incisions—has been described by Lever and Dahan.[26] In that technique, a second opposite penetrating clear corneal incision is placed over the steep meridian 180 degrees away from the main phaco incision. This approach is technically simple and requires no ancillary instrumentation; however, a second substantial penetrating incision is now present, possibly increasing the risk of wound leak or infection. In addition, single-plane, beveled incisions are known not to be as effective (for a given arc length) as more conventional perpendicular relaxing incisions for flattening the cornea.[20,27] Dr. Richard Mackool makes use of a similar technique that he refers to as double-penetrating LRIs.[28]

A distinctly different alternative for the correction of astigmatism is to utilize laser technology. Femtosecond laser-assisted relaxing incisions will be addressed in detail in Chapter 7. Excimer laser surgery is an important nonincisional approach for correcting astigmatism, which is often referred to as "bioptics," and is a technique first reported to address residual refractive error following implantation of myopic phakic IOLs, but it is useful in the setting of pseudophakic lens surgery as well.[29-31] In Zaldivar's original description, a laser in situ keratomileusis (LASIK) flap was created prior to the phakic implant procedure, and then, as necessary, the flap was lifted and the residual refractive error was corrected with the laser.[29] Today, most surgeons prefer to perform both the flap creation and the laser ablation concurrently following refractive lens surgery only as needed as an enhancement procedure, rather than as a primary approach to astigmatism management. In the author's experience, LASIK may be performed safely following IOL surgery within several weeks of the primary lens procedure, after refractive stability has been documented. Photorefractive keratectomy (PRK) is particularly well suited for this older pseudophakic population, which typically has only modest amounts of residual refractive error and has a higher incidence of dry eye and corneal surface problems. Custom wavefront-guided ablation may also be considered, as the pseudophakic eye no longer has a dynamic lens component, although obtaining a reliable wavefront aberrometry reading may be difficult with some lens designs, such as refractive multifocal optics.[32] For most refractive cataract surgeons, bioptics has become an integral part of the preoperative discussion with the patient, and, in the author's experience, its use is required in approximately 10% of cases, depending on the magnitude of the patient's preoperative refractive error (see Chapter 5 for further discussion). Although of limited popularity, conductive keratoplasty used in an off-label fashion has also been described as a means by which residual hyperopia and hyperopic astigmatism may be effectively reduced following cataract surgery.[33]

Finally, residual postoperative astigmatism, similar to residual spherical error, may be addressed by the implantation into the ciliary sulcus of a secondary low-power IOL. Such implants are now available internationally and may be available in the United States in the future.[34]

Limbal Relaxing Incisions

The first systematic study of the astigmatic effect of nonpenetrating incisions placed near the limbus dates back to 1898 and is credited to the Dutch ophthalmologist L.J. Lans.[35] Although the use of toric IOLs is increasing, LRIs have historically been the most common means by which surgeons address pre-existing astigmatism at the time of implant surgery.[36] Although the author's preference is to utilize a temporal, single-plane clear corneal phaco incision, one may utilize LRIs with any type of cataract incision, as long as the astigmatic effect is known and factored into the surgical plan. LRIs offer several advantages over astigmatic incisions placed within the more central cornea at smaller optical zones. First, one finds that LRIs' effect is more likely to take place in the intended corneal meridian, with less chance of causing a shift in the resultant cylinder axis. This presumably is due to a diminishing need for exact centration over the steep meridian using a more peripheral approach. Perhaps more important, there is less of a tendency to cause irregular corneal flattening, and hence, less chance of inducing irregular astigmatism. Technically, LRIs are easier to perform and more forgiving than shorter and more central corneal astigmatic incisions, and patients generally report less discomfort. Another important advantage gained by moving out to the limbus involves the "coupling ratio," which describes the amount of flattening that occurs in the incised meridian relative to the amount of steepening that results 90 degrees away. In the author's experience, paired LRIs (when kept at or under 90 degrees of arc length) exhibit a consistent 1:1 ratio; therefore, little change in the spheroequivalent is elicited, obviating the need to make any change in implant power.

Admittedly, these more peripheral incisions are less powerful, but they are still capable of correcting up to 3.00 to 4.00 D of astigmatism in the cataract-age population. One must keep in mind that the goal is to reduce the patient's cylinder, without overcorrecting or shifting the resultant axis. To achieve a given amount of correction, these peripheral intralimbal incisions must be longer in total arc length than the more centrally placed corneal astigmatic incisions. However, unlike longer radial keratotomy incisions, the peripheral incisions appear to be stable with regard to refractive effect, and they infrequently induce problems, such as dry eye syndrome or other pejorative effects from corneal denervation, although one must be cautious in eyes that are predisposed to such problems.[23,37] Their stability may be due to the proximity of well-vascularized limbal tissue, as well as the differing histologic tissue pattern that exists at this intralimbal location, compared with the central cornea. There are, of course, potential complications with any surgical technique and these are addressed in the sections that follow.

The Plan

Perhaps the most challenging aspect of astigmatism surgery involves the determination of the quantity and exact location of the cylinder that is to be corrected, thereby formulating a surgical plan (refer to Chapter 2 for a detailed discussion). Traditionally, most authors have recommended correcting astigmatism based on corneal measurements only, assuming any other refractive components would be lenticular in nature and eliminated by lens extraction. However, the author has found that it is helpful to study as many preoperative parameters as possible. Unfortunately, such preoperative measurements—keratometry, refraction, corneal topography, and newer modalities such as the Pentacam (Oculus)—do not always correlate. Lenticular astigmatism may account for some of this disparity, particularly in cases where there is a wide variance between refraction and corneal measurements; however, some discrepancies are likely, due to the inherent shortcomings of traditional measurements of astigmatism. Standard keratometry, for example, measures only 2 points in each meridian at a single optical zone of approximately 3 mm. The posterior corneal curvature and pupillary diameter may also affect measures of astigmatism and its impact on visual function.[38,39]

When confounding measurements do arise, one may compromise and average the disparate readings. For example, if a refraction shows 2.00 D of astigmatism and keratometry reveals only 1.00 D, it would be reasonable to correct for 1.25 to 1.50 D, especially if the cataract is not too dense and the refraction is reasonably reliable or if it is based on a historical refraction that was obtained prior to cataract formation. Alternatively, if preoperative calculations vary widely, one may defer placing the relaxing incisions until a stable refraction is obtained postimplantation, and any remaining astigmatism can be then corrected as needed. Limbal relaxing incisions may be safely performed in the office in an appropriate treatment-room setting or, in some surgeon's hands, even at the slit lamp. Corneal topography is increasingly becoming the overall guiding measurement on which the surgical plan is based. Topography is also helpful in detecting subtle corneal pathology, such as forme fruste keratoconus, which would likely negate the use of LRIs or subtle irregular astigmatism caused by epithelial basement membrane dystrophy, which might require a separate treatment plan.

Nomograms

When the amount of astigmatism to be corrected has been determined, a nomogram must be consulted to determine the appropriate arc length of the incisions. A number of popular nomograms are currently available.[40] As mentioned previously, the author's nomogram of choice originated from the work of Dr. Stephen Hollis and incorporates the concepts taught by Spencer Thornton, MD,[20] particularly his age modifiers (Table 3-1). After accounting for surgically induced cylinder from one's phaco and IOL incision, and assessing as many preoperative measurements as possible to determine the amount and location of the cylinder to be corrected, one would consult the appropriate section of the nomogram. With-the-rule astigmatism is considered to be from 45 to 135 degrees, and against-the-rule astigmatism is from 0 to 44 degrees or 136 to 180 degrees, as the arc length of the incisions differs somewhat based on this distinction. One then aligns the patient's age with the amount of preoperative cylinder to be corrected and finds the suggested arc length that the incisions should subtend.

An empiric blade depth setting is commonly used when performing LRIs, typically at 600 µm. This would seem to be a reasonable practice when treating cataract patients; however, in the setting of refractive lens exchange surgery or when utilizing presbyopia-correcting IOLs—where ultimate precision is required—it is the author's strong preference to perform peripheral pachymetry and use adjusted blade depth settings. Pachymetry may be performed either preoperatively or at the time of surgery. Readings are taken over the entire arc length of the intended incision, and an adjustable micrometer diamond blade is set to approximately 90% of the thinnest reading obtained. Refinements to the blade depth setting, as well as nomogram adjustments, may be necessary, depending on the individual surgeon's technique, the instruments used, and, in particular, the style of the blade. It is highly suggested that a diamond knife specifically designed for LRIs be used, as the quality and precision of the blade will greatly influence one's results. It should also be noted that in eyes that have previously undergone radial keratotomy, the length of the incisions should be reduced by approximately 50%, and in eyes that have undergone "significant" prior keratotomy surgery, it may be best to avoid additional incisional surgery and use a toric IOL or laser technology instead.

Paired incisions are preferred to optimize symmetric corneal flattening and are expressed in degrees of arc, rather than chord length. This is done to diminish over- and undercorrections for unusually small or large corneas, as corneal diameter may significantly impact the relative length of the arcuate incision and its resultant effect (Figure 3-1). Incisions are usually symmetric and orthogonal unless reliable topography strongly suggests asymmetric astigmatism. Irregular astigmatism, as seen in forms of keratoconus, may lead to unpredictable results when treated with relaxing incisions and is likely better managed by using other modalities.

Table 3-1. The "NAPA" Nomogram: Nichamin Age & Pachymetry-Adjusted Intralimbal Arcuate Astigmatic Nomogram

WITH-THE-RULE ASTIGMATISM (STEEP AXIS 45 TO 135 DEGREES)

Preoperative Cylinder (Diopters)	*Paired Incisions in Degrees of Arc*					
	20 to 30 yo	*31 to 40 yo*	*41 to 50 yo*	*51 to 60 yo*	*61 to 70 yo*	*71 to 80 yo*
0.75	40	35	35	30	30	
1.00	45	40	40	35	35	30
1.25	55	50	45	40	35	35
1.50	60	55	50	45	40	40
1.75	65	60	55	50	45	45
2.00	70	65	60	55	50	45
2.25	75	70	65	60	55	50
2.50	80	75	70	65	60	55
2.75	85	80	75	70	65	60
3.00	90	90	85	80	70	65

AGAINST-THE-RULE ASTIGMATISM (STEEP AXIS 0 TO 44 DEGREES/136 TO 180 DEGREES)

Preoperative Cylinder (Diopters)	*Paired Incisions in Degrees of Arc*					
	20 to 30 yo	*31 to 40 yo*	*41 to 50 yo*	*51 to 60 yo*	*61 to 70 yo*	*71 to 80 yo*
0.75	45	40	40	35	35	30
1.00	50	45	45	40	40	35
1.25	55	55	50	45	40	35
1.50	60	60	55	50	45	40
1.75	65	65	60	55	50	45
2.00	70	70	65	60	55	50
2.25	75	75	70	65	60	55
2.50	80	80	75	70	65	60
2.75	85	85	80	75	70	65
3.00	90	90	85	80	75	70

Blade depth setting is at 90% of the thinnest pachymetry.

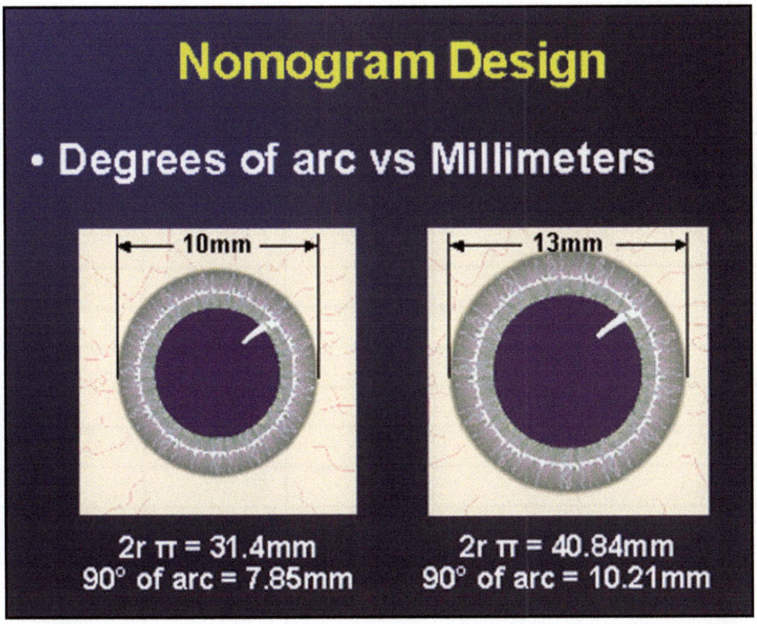

Figure 3-1. Nomogram designs. Note the relative disparity in incision length between a large and small corneal diameter, if measured in millimeters. Degrees of arc lend consistency, irrespective of corneal size.

The emerging field of femtosecond laser-assisted cataract surgery will surely prove to be a revolutionary advance in many ways, not the least of which will be in the "automation" of our astigmatic relaxing incisions. Chapter 7 is dedicated to this subject, although Table 3-2 in this chapter also provides the author's adjusted LRI nomogram for use with the femtosecond laser, with incision placement at the 9.0-mm optical zone. Current-generation femtosecond lasers cannot always image the most peripheral intralimbal tissue well, particularly if there is a significant arcus senilis present. As such, most laser-assisted incisions are placed at approximately the 9.0-mm optical zone. If the laser relaxing incisions are placed at a larger optical zone, then the nomogram may need to be adjusted for slightly longer arcuate lengths; the opposite is true if a smaller optical zone is utilized. Also, if sub-Bowman's layer incisions or intrastromal incisions are created without penetration through the corneal epithelium, less effect will be seen, at least until the epithelium is later opened and the incisions are spread apart. This latter technique can be a helpful way in which the effect of laser LRIs may be titrated in the early postoperative period.

Surgical Technique

Some surgeons prefer to perform LRIs at the conclusion of surgery in the event that a complication occurs necessitating a modification to the phaco incision. However, the author's preference for routine cases is to place these relaxing incisions at the outset of surgery to minimize epithelial disruption. The exception to this rule occurs in the case where the phaco incision will intersect or be superimposed upon an LRI of greater than 40 degrees of arc length. For a surgeon utilizing a temporal clear corneal phaco incision, this would occur when correcting for a moderately high amount of ATR astigmatism. In such a case, if the temporal relaxing incision was to be extended to its full arc length at the start of surgery, significant gaping and edema may result, secondary to intraoperative wound manipulation. To avoid this potential problem, the temporal incision is first made by creating a 2-plane, deeply grooved phaco incision (the depth being based on pachymetry, as noted previously, and the arc length is determined by the implant being used). Later, just prior to the lens implantation, with a firm viscoelastic-filled eye, the partial relaxing incision is extended to its full arc length as dictated by the nomogram. The keratome entry, when fashioning this combined, or superimposed, LRI and phaco tunnel, is best achieved by pressing the bottom surface

Table 3-2. Nichamin Femtosecond—LRI Nomogram

WITH-THE-RULE ASTIGMATISM (STEEP AXIS 45 TO 135 DEGREES)

Preoperative Cylinder (Diopters)	*Paired Incisions in Degrees of Arc*					
	20 to 30 yo	*31 to 40 yo*	*41 to 50 yo*	*51 to 60 yo*	*61 to 70 yo*	*71 to 80 yo*
0.75	39	34	30	27	25	23
1.00	44	39	35	33	31	28
1.25	50	45	41	38	35	33
1.50	55	51	47	43	40	37
1.75	60	56	52	48	44	41
2.00	65	60	56	52	48	45
2.25	70	64	60	56	52	48
2.50	75	69	64	60	56	52
2.75	80	73	68	64	60	56
3.00	85	78	73	69	65	60

AGAINST-THE-RULE ASTIGMATISM (STEEP AXIS 0 TO 44 DEGREES/136 TO 180 DEGREES)

Preoperative Cylinder (Diopters)	*Paired Incisions in Degrees of Arc*					
	20 to 30 yo	*31 to 40 yo*	*41 to 50 yo*	*51 to 60 yo*	*61 to 70 yo*	*71 to 80 yo*
0.75	40	35	31	28	26	25
1.00	46	41	38	36	33	31
1.25	52	48	45	41	37	35
1.50	58	54	50	46	42	39
1.75	63	59	55	51	47	43
2.00	67	63	59	55	51	47
2.25	71	67	63	59	55	51
2.50	75	71	67	63	59	55
2.75	80	75	71	67	63	59
3.00	85	79	75	71	67	63

Approximate 9.0-mm optical zone, 85% depth.

of the keratome blade downward on the outer or posterior edge of the partial LRI. The keratome is then advanced into the LRI at an iris-parallel plane. This angulation will promote a dissection that takes place at a midstromal depth, which will help assure adequate tunnel length and a self-sealing closure.

Proper centration of the incisions over the steep corneal meridian is of utmost importance. Increasing evidence supports the notion that significant cyclotorsion may occur when assuming a supine position.[41] Classic teaching states that an axis deviation of only 15 degrees may result in

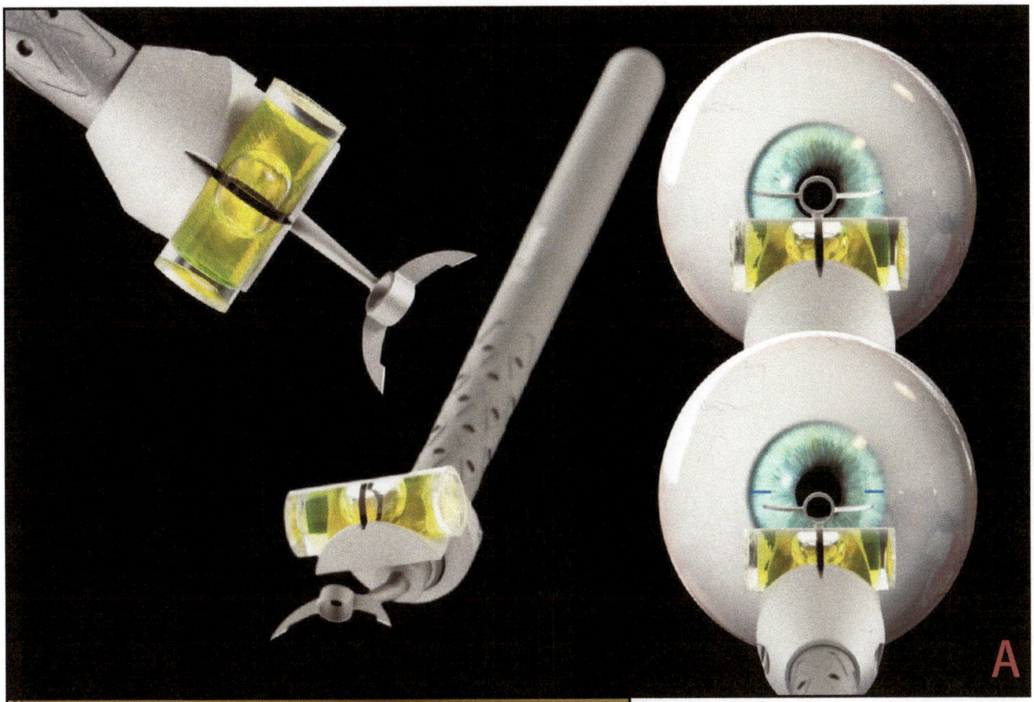

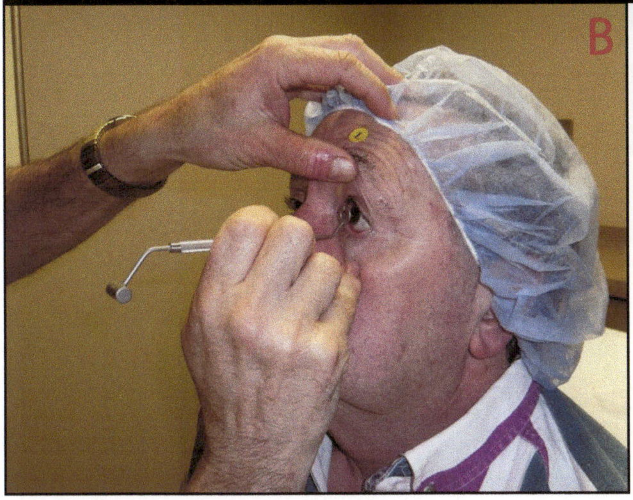

Figure 3-2. (A) Corneal marker with bubble level for placement of meridional orientation marks (Mastel Precision). (Reprinted with permission from Mastel Precision.) (B) Upright patient receiving corneal orientation marks prior to surgery. (From Tasman W, Jaeger EA, eds. *Duane's Ophthalmology 2011*. Lippincott Williams and Wilkins; 2011. Reprinted with permission.)

a 50% reduction of surgical effect.[5] This reduction in effect holds true for both relaxing incisions and toric IOLs. For this reason, an orientation mark(s) is placed at the patient's limbus while he or she is in an upright position. This is particularly important when using injection anesthesia where unpredictable ocular rotation may occur. The author prefers placing multiple radial marks using a dedicated marking instrument to assure proper orientation (Figure 3-2). Some surgeons prefer to place their orientation mark with the patient seated at the slit lamp, thereby achieving better control and higher magnification. Newer digital reference and guidance instruments are being designed to further improve and facilitate this critical orientation step[42] (Figure 3-3).

An additional measure that may be used to help center the relaxing incisions is to identify the steep meridian (plus cylinder) intraoperatively, using some form of keratoscopy. The steep meridian over which the incisions are to be placed should correspond to the shorter diameter of the reflected corneal mire. A simple, handheld device such as the Maloney keratoscope (Bausch

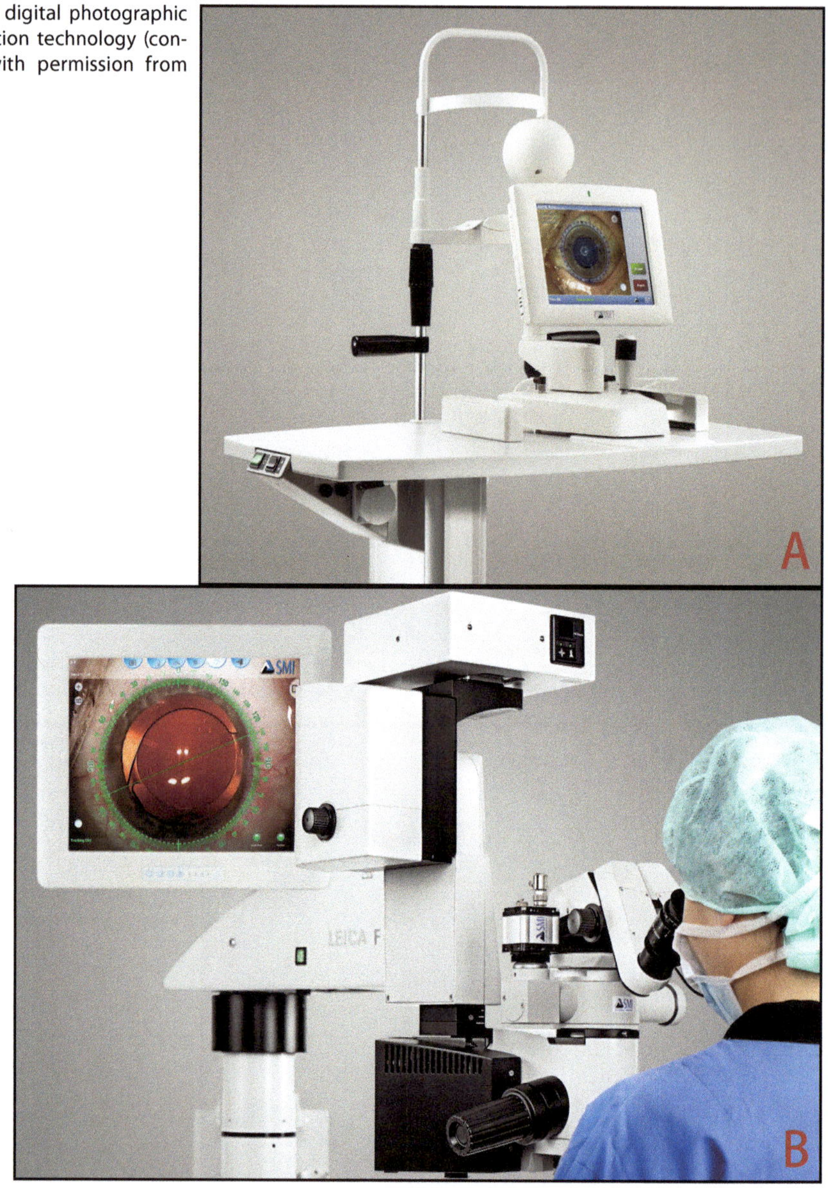

Figure 3-3. (A-D) SMI digital photographic reference and orientation technology (continued). (Reprinted with permission from SMI.)

& Lomb Storz, and Katena Products Inc) or the Nichamin keratoscope (Mastel Precision) works well, or a more robust and well-defined mire may be obtained through a microscope-mounted instrument such as the Mastel illuminating surgical keratoscope (Mastel Precision) (Figure 3-4). Recently, intraoperative wavefront aberrometry has become commercially available, which may further help to guide both the positioning and length of the relaxing incisions, allowing for real-time refinements during the actual surgical procedure. This device is also used to aid in the meridional positioning of toric IOLs and can be used to affirm proper spherical power selection of an implanted IOL[43,44] (Figure 3-5).

One then utilizes a Mendez ring (Mastel Precision) or a similar degree gauge that, when aligned with the limbal orientation mark(s), yields the desired meridian over which the incisions are to be centered (Figure 3-6). The extent of arc to be incised may be demarcated in several different ways. Various press-on markers are available, such as Rhein Medical Inc's Dell-Nichamin marker

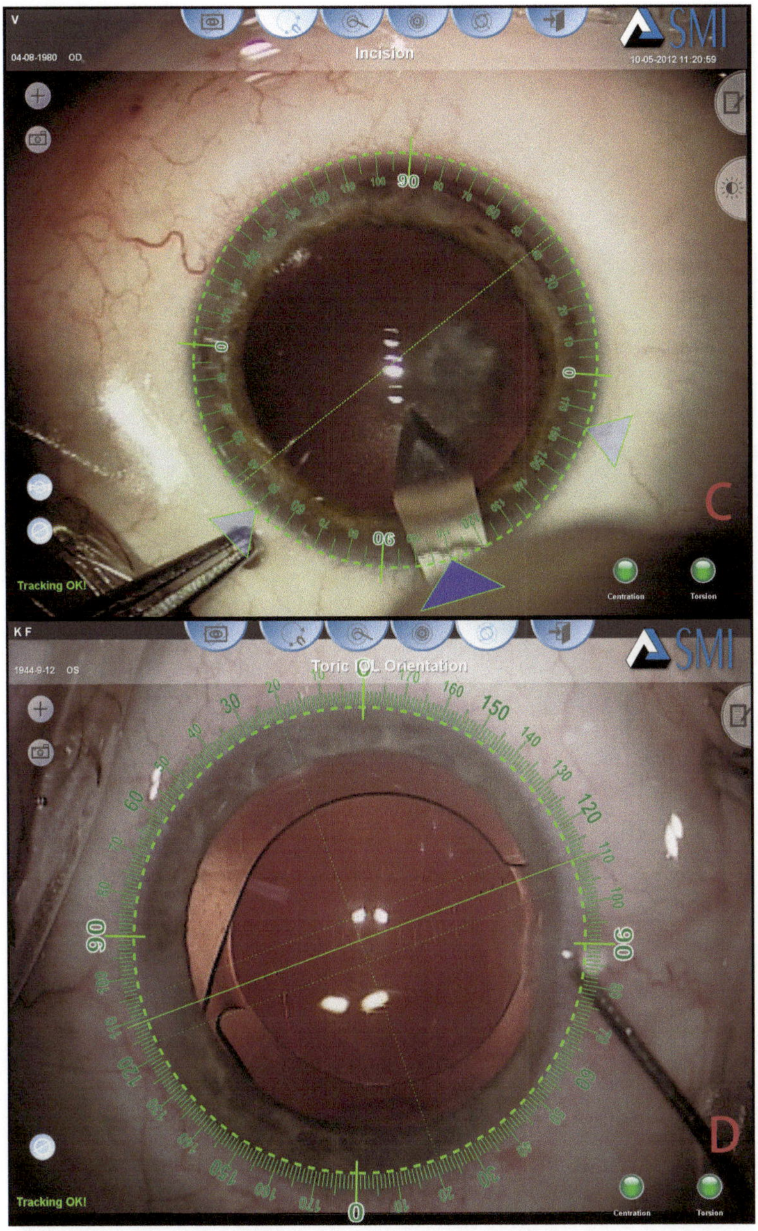

Figure 3-3 (continued). (A-D) SMI digital photographic reference and orientation technology. (Reprinted with permission from SMI.)

(Figure 3-7). The author's current preferred method uses an engraved ring that is centered over the steep meridian, and its surface markings delineate the arc length to be incised (Figure 3-8). Ink marks may be placed on the corneal surface, delineated by this ring, showing the start and end points of the relaxing incision (Figure 3-9).

The LRI should be placed at the most peripheral extent of the clear corneal tissue, just inside of the true surgical limbus. This holds true, irrespective of the presence of pannus or blood vessels. If bleeding occurs, it may be ignored and will cease spontaneously. One must avoid placing the incisions further out at the true surgical limbus, in that a significant reduction of effect will likely occur due to both an increased tissue thickness and a variation in tissue composition; these incisions are, therefore, truly intralimbal in nature. In creating the incision, it is important to hold the knife perpendicular to the corneal surface to achieve consistent depth and effect. Good hand and

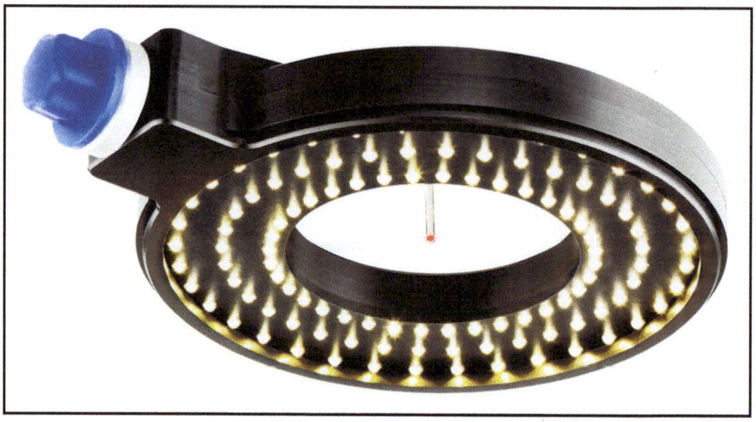

Figure 3-4. Mastel Precision's illuminating surgical keratoscope. (Reprinted with permission from Mastel Precision.)

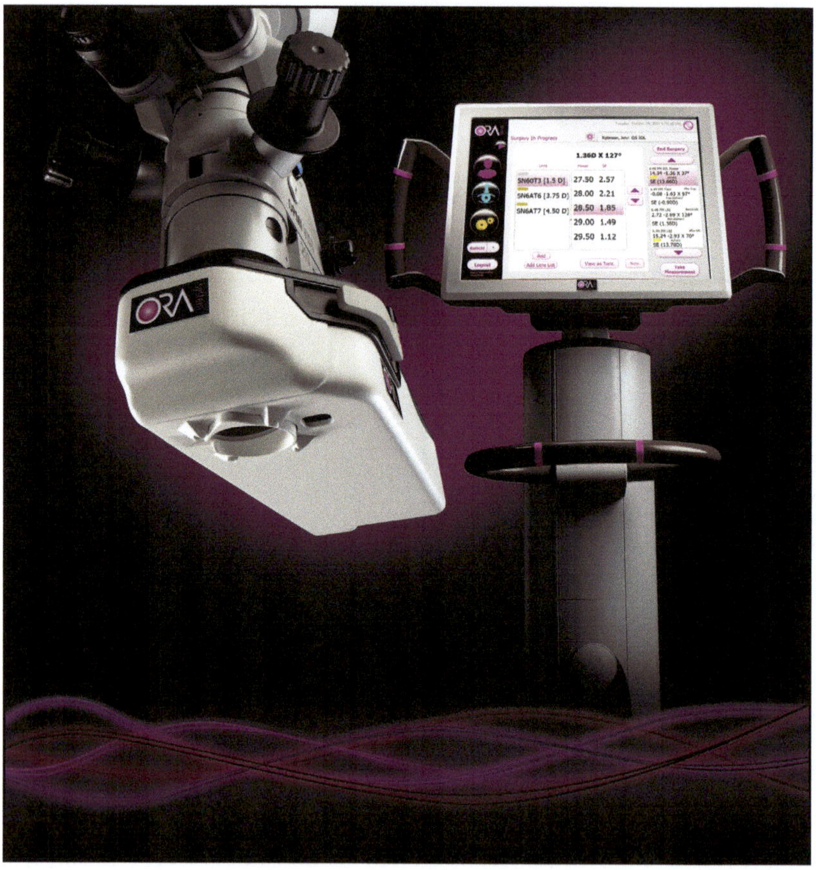

Figure 3-5. WaveTec Vision's ORA intraoperative wavefront aberrometer. (From Tasman W, Jaeger EA, eds. *Duane's Ophthalmology 2011.* Lippincott Williams and Wilkins; 2011. Reprinted with permission.)

wrist support is important, and the blade should be held as if one were throwing a dart, such that the instrument may be rotated between the thumb and index finger as it is being advanced, leading to smooth arcuate incisions. Typically, the right hand is used to create incisions on the right side of the globe, and the left hand is used for incisions on the left side. In most cases, it is more efficient to pull the blade toward oneself, as opposed to pushing it away. A lightly moistened corneal surface will help to prevent epithelial disruption, but this may mask an unintentional perforation.

Adequate exposure of the perilimbal region is important to allow for perpendicularity between the corneal surface and the diamond blade. As such, a locking-lid speculum is helpful and is

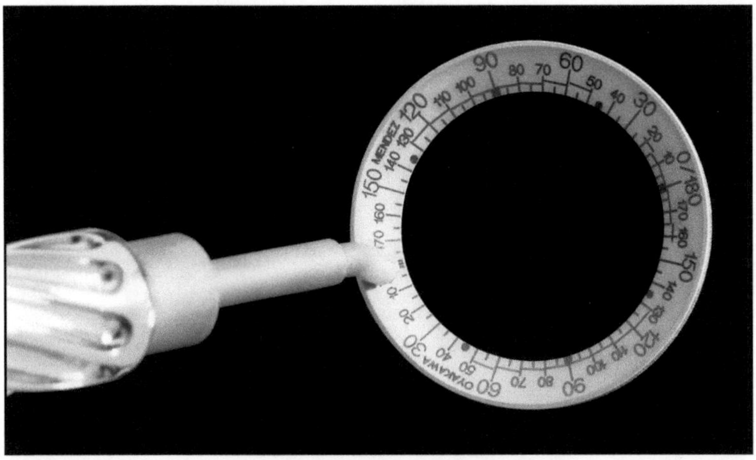

Figure 3-6. Mendez ring (Mastel Precision) used to locate the steep corneal meridian based on preplaced orientation marks. (Reprinted with permission from Mastel Precision.)

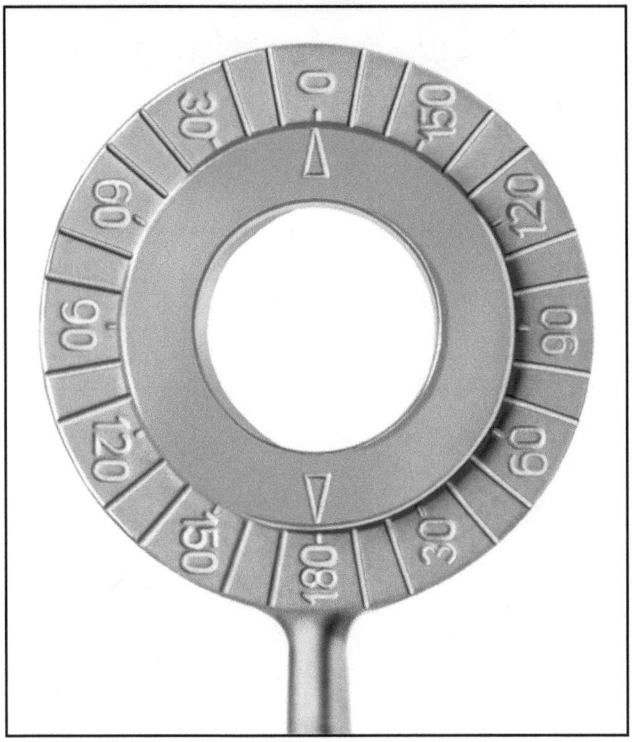

Figure 3-7. Dell-Nichamin marker (Rhein Medical Inc) may be used to mark both the central steep meridian and the intended arc length of the incisions. (From Tasman W, Jaeger EA, eds. *Duane's Ophthalmology 2011*. Lippincott Williams and Wilkins; 2011. Reprinted with permission.)

further facilitated through the use of a modified Fine-Thornton fixation ring—the Nichamin fixation ring and gauge, available from Mastel Precision, Bausch & Lomb Storz, and Rhein Medical Inc—that aids in moving the globe into an optimal position for creation of the relaxing incision. This fixation ring also assists in verifying the arc length of the incision by virtue of 10-degree incremental radial marks on the surface of the ring (Figure 3-10).

As noted, in the setting of concomitant cataract surgery, an empiric blade depth setting of 600 μm has been traditionally used. More recently, adjusted blade depth settings, based on pachymetry, are favored for optimal precision. Various knives have been designed specifically for this application, ranging from disposable steel blades to exquisite gemstone diamond knives. Synthetic diamond materials are also available and vary in quality from nearly perfect, single crystal materials that rival natural occurring gemstones (but they are often yellow in color) to

Figure 3-8. Jarvi/Olson arcuate ring guide (Mastel Precision) used to mark the arc length of the relaxing incisions. (Reprinted with permission from Mastel Precision.)

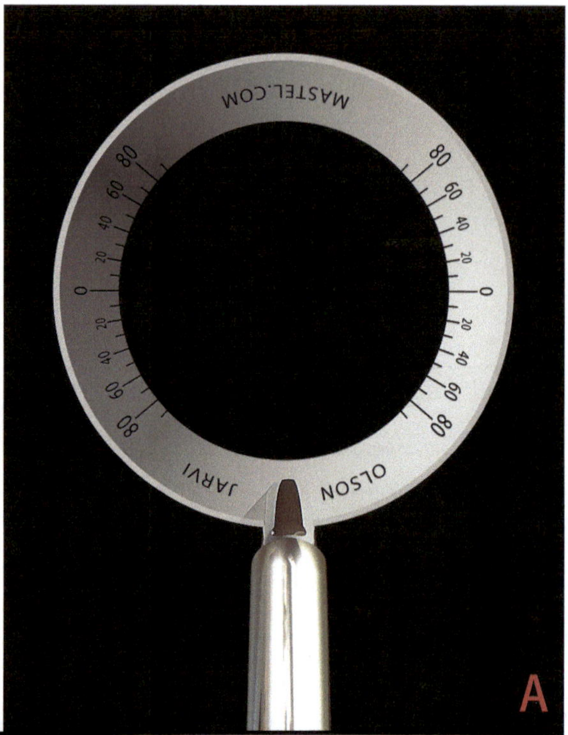

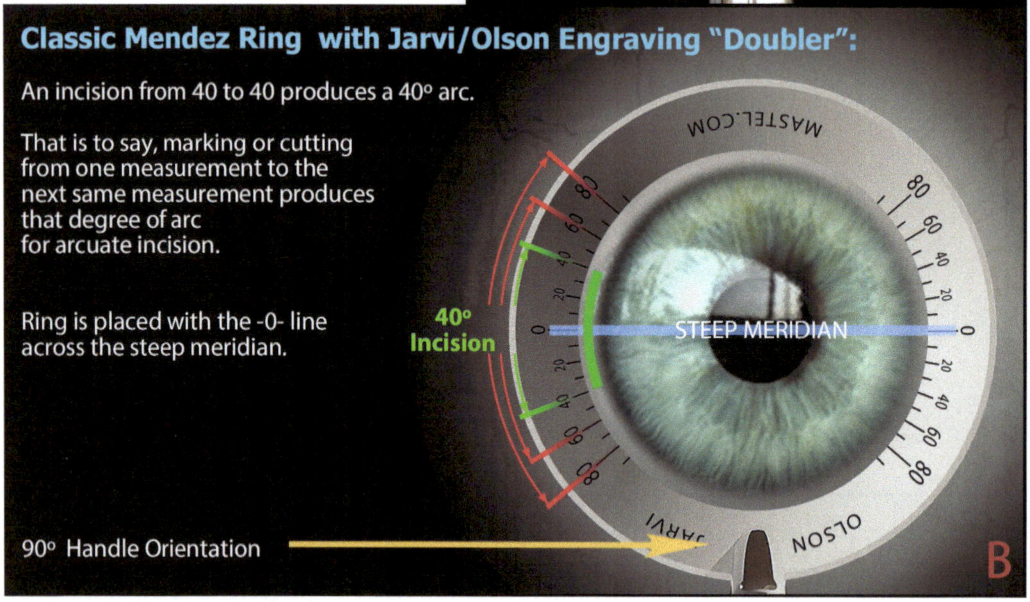

less expensive polycrystal-fused materials that are typically less durable and whose edges are laser cut, which may yield less precise cutting characteristics. Some of these less expensive designs are intended for limited reuse. The author's preference is for high-quality diamond blade technology, which incorporates a single small and arced footplate for enhanced visualization at the limbus. Two such models, one with a preset depth of 600 µm and the other with an adjustable micrometer handle, are made by Mastel Precision (Figure 3-11). Similar designs are available from Bausch & Lomb Storz, Rhein Medical, ASICO LLC, and other manufacturers.

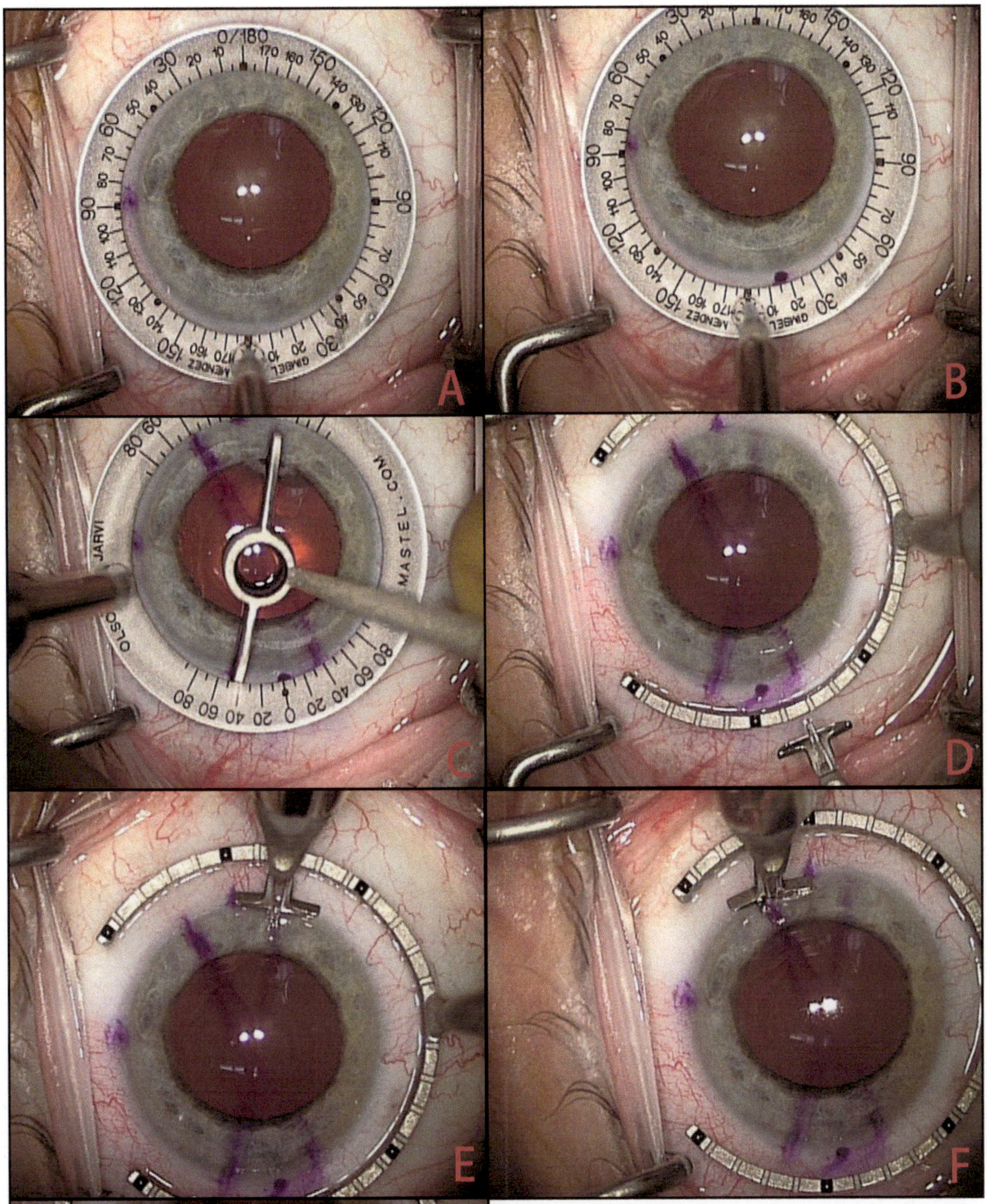

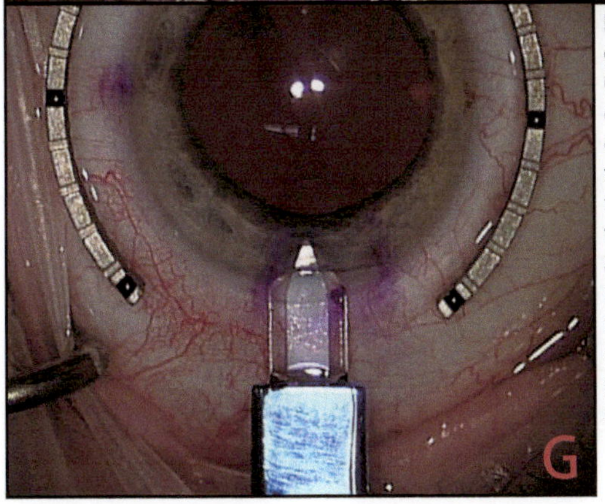

Figure 3-9. (A) 90-degree reference mark of Mendez gauge aligned with 6 o'clock limbal orientation ink mark. (B) Additional mark placed at the steep 15-degree meridian over which relaxing incisions will be centered. (C) Two-ray corneal marker is used in conjunction with Jarvi/Olson ring to delineate the extent of arc to be incised. (D) Nichamin fixation ring placed outside of limbus to optimally position the globe. Note the black hash mark on the ring is aligned with the steep meridian, and the 10-degree radial marks may be further used to delineate the arc length of the incision. (E) Nasal LRI started. (F) Nasal LRI completed. (G) Keratome placed through temporal LRI to compete the phaco incision. (Reprinted with permission from Wolters Kluwer.)

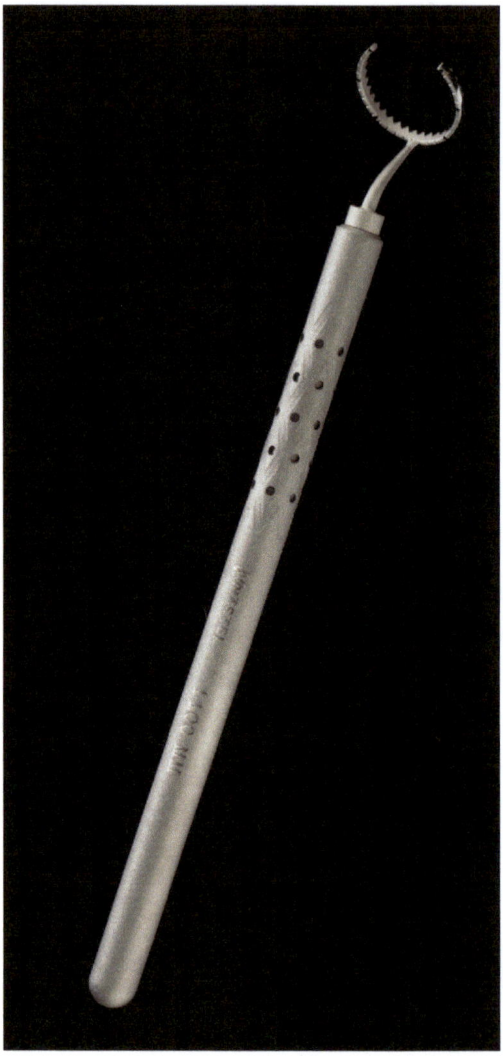

Figure 3-10. Nichamin-modified Fine-Thornton fixation ring (Mastel Precision). (Reprinted with permission of Mastel Precision.)

Increased Comfort for Patient and Physician

Interestingly, foreign body sensation is one of the most common patient complaints following contemporary phaco surgery. Intralimbal relaxing incisions, compared to more central corneal incisions (smaller optical zones), improve patient comfort. A lightly moistened corneal surface will help to prevent epithelial disruption, but this may mask an unintentional perforation—a very rare event that can occur with proper technique and instrumentation. If epithelial drag is seen to occur during surgery, it is best to stop and exit the incision, then reenter the incision and continue advancing the blade in gradual increments, thus avoiding the stripping of a large sheet of epithelium.

With the addition of a postoperative topical nonsteroidal anti-inflammatory drug, patient comfort is quite acceptable, and topical lubricants are further used as needed. Upon examination, these incisions appear to heal quickly and are nearly unidentifiable within several days. The astigmatic effect is generally stable within days to weeks postoperatively, depending on the arcuate length of the incisions.

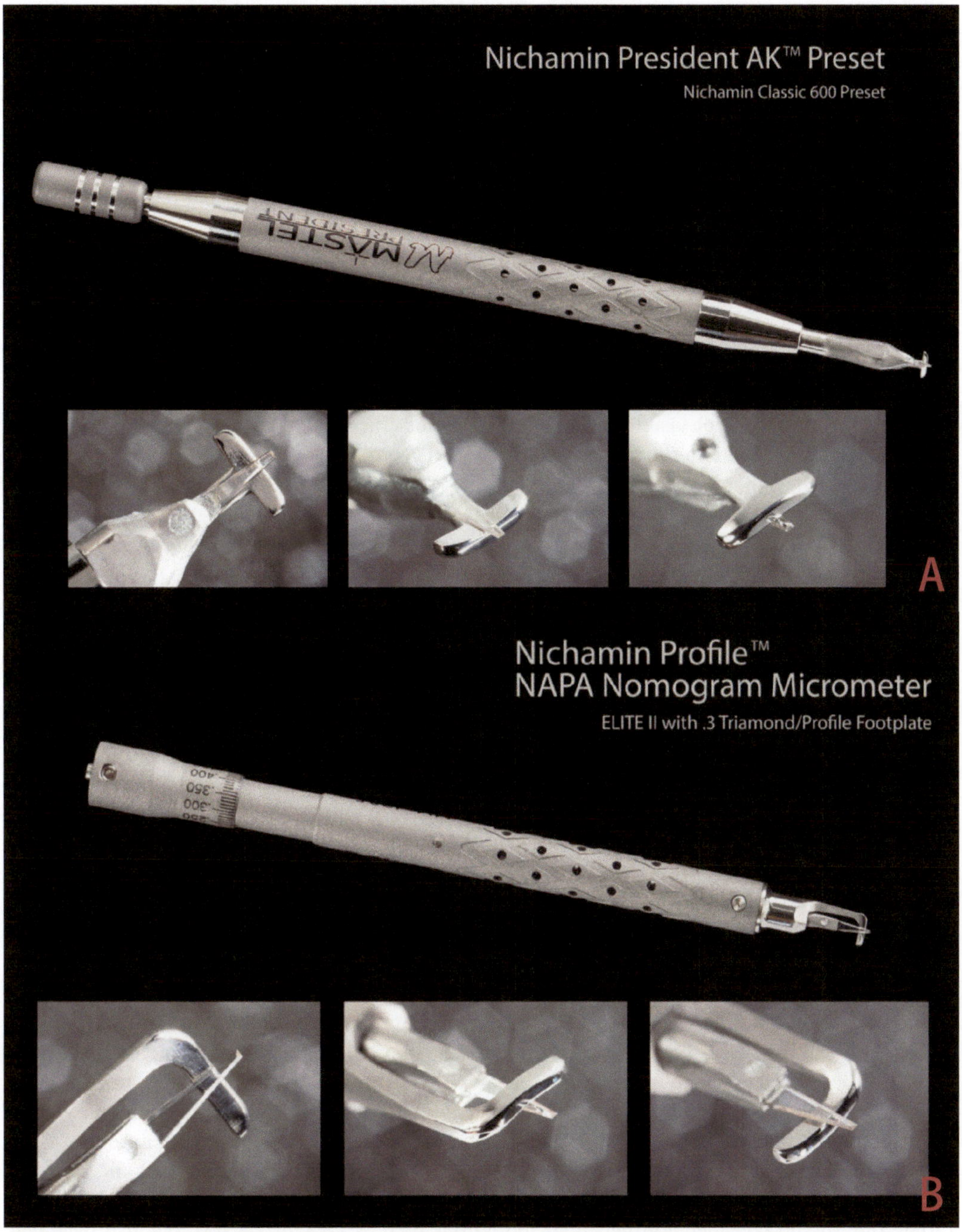

Figure 3-11. (A) LRI diamond blade with preset depth of 600 μm (Mastel Precision). (B) LRI diamond blade with adjustable depth micrometer (Mastel Precision). (Reprinted with permission of Mastel Precision.)

Complications

As discussed, LRIs are proving to be a safer and more forgiving approach to managing astigmatism, compared with more central corneal incisions. Nonetheless, as with any surgical technique, potential complications exist, and several are listed in Table 3-3. Of these, the most likely to be encountered is the placement of incisions on the wrong axis. When this occurs, it typically takes

Table 3-3. Potential Problems	
Infection	Induced irregular astigmatism
Weakening of the globe	Misalignment/axis shift
Perforation	Wound gape and discomfort
Decreased corneal sensation	Operating upon the wrong (opposite) axis!

the form of a 90-degree error with positioning on the opposite, flat meridian. This, of course, results in an increase and the likely doubling of the patient's pre-existing cylinder. Compulsive attention is required in this regard. The surgeon ought to consider using safety checks to prevent this frustrating complication from occurring, such as having a written plan that is brought into the operating room and is kept visible and properly oriented. Incisions are always placed on the plus (+) cylinder axis, opposite to the minus (-) cylinder axis.

Corneal perforation is possible, although it is rare when utilizing a blade depth determined by pachymetry measurements or an empiric setting of 600 µm. Corneal perforation may be due to improper setting of the blade depth or as a result of a defect in the micrometer mechanism. This latter problem may arise after repeated autoclaving and many sterilization runs. Periodic inspection and calibration is therefore warranted, even with preset, single-depth knives. When encountered, unlike radial microperforations, these circumferential perforations will rarely self-seal and will likely require placement of temporary sutures (for further discussion of complications related to the use of LRIs, see Chapter 6).

Enhancement Techniques

As mentioned previously, LRIs lend themselves well to in-office "touch-ups." Although some surgeons will place or extend incisions at the slit lamp, it is the author's preference to use a small operating microscope and to perform the procedure within a dedicated treatment room. In the author's experience, this provides better surgical control, as well as increased patient comfort. In the case of residual astigmatism without prior incisional correction, one uses the same technique and nomogram as described.

In the case of an undercorrection following previous LRIs, one should inspect the length and positioning of the incisions. As previously indicated, placement of the incisions too far out into the true surgical limbus and beyond the clear cornea will often lead to undercorrection. If the arc length and location appear to be adequate, one should suspect that the patient has an unusually thick cornea. This occurs most frequently in hyperopic eyes. In this situation, pachymetry should be performed and the incisions may be redeepened or extended. When faced with an overcorrection, one should resist the temptation to place additional incisions in a new meridian. This can lead to an unstable cornea with unpredictable refractive results, or worse, induce irregular astigmatism. Rather, one should consider nonincisional modalities such as PRK or LASIK. We also have had reasonable results in this setting using off-label conductive keratoplasty, particularly if the overcorrection involves hyperopic astigmatism.[32] As mentioned previously, secondary low-power piggyback IOLs are also an option (currently not available in the United States), especially if further corneal surgery is contraindicated.[34]

To correct unusually high levels of astigmatism, LRIs may be used in conjunction with a toric IOL or excimer laser surgery (bioptics). In several rare cases, the author has combined all 3 modalities and safely corrected up to 9.00 D of pre-existing astigmatism!

Conclusion

Success following modern implant surgery is increasingly defined by the refractive outcome that is achieved, and management of pre-existing astigmatism is an integral component and determinant of patient satisfaction. Although toric implants and advanced laser technologies are serving to further advance the field of refractive IOL surgery, manual LRIs continue to be an extraordinarily useful and requisite technique. Fortunately, their use and mastery fall well within the purview of all contemporary implant surgeons.

References

1. Brick DC. Risk management lessons from a review of 168 cataract surgery claims. *Surv Ophthalmol.* 1999:43(4):356-360.
2. 2009 survey of US ASCRS members. Analeyz, Inc. http://www.analeyz.com/Analeyz%20ASCRS%202009.htm. Accessed September 28, 2010.
3. Findl O, Drexler W, Menapace R, Hitzenberger CK, Fercher AF. High precision biometry of pseudophakic eyes using partial coherence interferometry. *J Cataract Refract Surg.* 1998:24(8):1087-1093.
4. [No author listed] Small incision surgery: wound construction and closure. *J Cataract Refract Surg.* 1991:17(suppl):659-748.
5. Abrams D. Ophthalmic optics and refraction. In: Duke-Elder SS, ed. *System of Ophthalmology.* St. Louis, MO: Mosby; 1970:671-674.
6. Buzard K, Shearing S, Relyea R. Incidence of astigmatism in a cataract practice. *J Refract Surg.* 1988;4:173.
7. Wallace RB. *Refractive Cataract Surgery and Multifocal IOLs.* Thorofare, NJ: SLACK Incorporated, 2000.
8. Novis C. Astigmatism and toric intraocular lenses. *Curr Opin Ophthalmol.* 2000;11(1):47-50.
9. Trindade F, Oliveira A, Frasson M. Benefit of against-the-rule astigmatism to uncorrected near acuity. *J Cataract Refract Surg.* 1997;23(1):82-85.
10. Savage H, Rothstein M, Davuluri G, El Ghormli L, Zaetta DM. Myopic astigmatism and presbyopia trial. *Am J Ophthalmol.* 2003;135(5):628-632.
11. Kobashi H, Kamiya K, Shimizu K, Kawamorita T, Uozato H. Effect of axis orientation on visual performance in astigmatic eyes. *J Cataract Refract Surg.* 2012;38(8):1352-1359.
12. Lyle WA, Jin G. Prospective evaluation of early visual and refractive effects with small clear corneal incisions for cataract surgery. *J Cataract Refract Surg.* 1996;22(10):1456-1460.
13. Masket S, Tennen DG. Astigmatic stabilization of 3.0mm temporal clear corneal cataract incisions. *J Cataract Refract Surg.* 1996;22(10):1451-1455.
14. Masket S, Wang L, Belani S. Induced astigmatism with 2.2- and 3.0-mm coaxial phacoemulsification incisions. *J Refract Surg.* 2009;25(1):21-24.
15. Sun XY, Vicary D, Montgomery P, Griffiths M. Toric intraocular lenses for correcting astigmatism in 130 eyes. *Ophthalmology.* 2000;107(9):1776-1781.
16. Nichamin LD. Combined technique: AK and LASIK. *J Cataract Refract Surg.* 2001;27(5):648-650.
17. Osher RH. *Combining phacoemulsification with corneal relaxing incisions for reduction of preexisting astigmatism.* Paper presented at: Annual meeting of the American Intraocular Implant Society; 1984; Los Angeles, CA.
18. Maloney WF. *Refractive cataract replacement: a comprehensive approach to maximize refractive benefits of cataract extraction.* Paper presented at: Annual Meeting of the American Society of Cataract and Refractive Surgery; 1986; Los Angeles, CA.
19. Osher RH. Transverse astigmatic keratotomy combined with cataract surgery. In: Thompson K, Waring G, eds. *Contemporary Refractive Surgery-Ophthalmology Clinics of North America.* Philadelphia, PA: W.B. Saunders Co; 1992:717-725.
20. Thornton SP. *Radial and Astigmatic Keratotomy: The American System of Precise, Predictable Refractive Surgery.* Thorofare, NJ: SLACK Incorporated; 1994.
21. Budak K, Friedman NF, Koch DD. Limbal relaxing incisions with cataract surgery. *J Cataract Refract Surg.* 1998;24(4):503-508.
22. Muller-Jensen K, Fischer P, Siepe U. Limbal relaxing incisions to correct astigmatism in clear corneal cataract surgery. *J Refract Surg.* 1999,15(5):586-589.
23. Nichamin LD. *Changing approach to astigmatism management during phacoemulsification: peripheral arcuate astigmatic relaxing incisions.* Paper presented at: Symposium on Cataract, IOL and Refractive Surgery, Congress on Ophthalmic Practice Management; May 20-24, 2000; Boston, MA.
24. Koch MJ, Kohnen T. Refractive cataract surgery. *Curr Opin Ophthalmol.* 1999;10(1):10-15.

25. Kaufmann C, Peter J, Ooi K, et al; Queen Elizabeth Astigmatism Study Group. Limbal relaxing incisions versus on-axis incisions to reduce corneal astigmatism at the time of cataract surgery. *J Cataract Refract Surg.* 2005;31(12):2261-2265.
26. Lever J, Dahan E. Opposite clear corneal incisions to correct preexisting astigmatism in cataract surgery. *J Cataract Refract Surg.* 2000, 26(6):803-805.
27. Nichamin LD. Opposite clear corneal incisions. *J Cataract Refract Surg.* 2001,27(1):7-8.
28. Caceres V. Reducing preexisting corneal astigmatism. *EyeWorld.* June 2011.
29. Zaldivar R, Davidorf JM, Oscerow S, Ricur G, Piezzi V. Combined posterior chamber phakic intraocular lens and laser in situ keratomileusis: bioptics for extreme myopia. *J Refract Surg.* 1999;15(3):299-308.
30. Nichamin LD. *Bioptics: expanding its role to pseudophakia.* Paper presented at: Symposium on Cataract, IOL and Refractive Surgery; June 1-5, 2002; Philadelphia, PA.
31. Nichamin LD. Expanding the role of bioptics to the pseudophakic patient. *J Cataract Refract Surg.* 2001;27(9):1343-1344.
32. Nichamin LD. Bioptics for the pseudophakic patient. In: Gills JP, ed. *A Complete Guide to Astigmatism Management: An Ophthalmic Manifesto.* Thorofare, NJ: SLACK Incorporated; 2003:37-39.
33. Nichamin LD. *Results of CK after cataract surgery.* Paper presented at: Symposium on Cataract, IOL and Refractive Surgery, Congress on Ophthalmic Practice Management; May 1-5, 2004; San Diego, CA.
34. Vyas, A, Naredran R, Bacon P. *Refractive outcome of piggy-back sulcus-fixated lens to correct residual ametropia and astigmatism.* Paper presented at: XXVIII Congress of the European Society of Cataract and Refractive Surgery; September 4-8, 2010; Paris, France.
35. Schimmelpfenning BH, Waring GO. Development of radial keratotomy in the nineteenth century. In: Waring GO, ed. *Refractive Keratotomy for Myopia and Astigmatism.* St. Louis, MO:Mosby-Year Book Inc; 1992:174-175.
36. Toric IOLs represent 7.5% of the market. *Market Scope;* 2012:Q2.
37. Donnenfeld ED, Holland EJ, Nichamin LD, et.al. *A multicenter evaluation of the effects of cataract extraction and limbal relaxing incisions on corneal sensation.* Poster presented at: Annual Meeting of the American Academy of Ophthalmology; October 24, 2011;Orlando, FL.
38. Koch DD. *Corneal optics for IOL selection: cracking the code.* Paper presented at: Annual Meeting of the American Society of Cataract and Refractive Surgery; April 20-24, 2012; Chicago, IL.
39. Visser N, Bauer NJ, Ruijts RM. Residual astigmatism following toric intraocular lens Implantation related to pupil size. *J Refract Surg.* 2012;28(10):729-732.
40. Gills JP. *A Complete Guide to Astigmatism Management.* Thorofare, NJ: SLACK Incorporated; 2003.
41. Swami AU, Steinert RF, Osborne WE, White AA. Rotational malposition during laser in situ keratomileusis. *Am J Ophthalmol.* 2002;133(4):561-562.
42. Nuijts RM, Viser N. *Assessment of cyclotorsion errors in marker-based toric IOL.* Paper presented at: Symposium on Cataract, IOL and Refractive Surgery, Congress on Ophthalmic Practice Management; April 9-14, 2010; Boston, MA.
43. Packer M. Effect of intraoperative aberrometry on the rate of postoperative enhancement: retrospective study. *J Cataract Refract Surg.* 2010;36(5):747-755.
44. Wiley W. *Reducing residual cylinder with toric IOLs guided by Orange®.* Program and abstracts of the Annual Meeting of the American Society of Cataract and Refractive Surgery; April 9-14, 2010; Boston, MA.

A version of Chapter 3 has been previously published in Tasman W, Jaeger EA, eds. *Duane's Ophthalmology 2011.* Philadelphia, PA: Lippincott Williams & Wilkins; 2011.

4

This Is How I Do It

Section 1: Limbal Relaxing Incisions to Correct Astigmatism

James P. Gills, MD and Pit Gills, MD

Historical Perspective

James P. Gills, MD

One of the most important areas of cataract surgery that I have focused on over the course of my career is the management of astigmatism. Early on, when I performed extracapsular cataract extraction, my goal was to avoid inducing astigmatism and to minimize it through the use of sutures. However, with the advent of phacoemulsification and the introduction of foldable intraocular lenses (IOLs), my attention turned from managing postoperative astigmatism to reducing pre-existing astigmatism. Today, the use of astigmatic keratotomy (whether performed manually or with the femtosecond laser) and the toric IOL allows us to treat our patients with greater precision than ever before, while providing the best quality vision of their lives.

Limbal Relaxing Incisions

Limbal relaxing incisions (LRIs) are one of the simplest, most cost-effective procedures available to reduce astigmatism. I coined this term years ago; however, it is not an ideal description of the procedure. To produce the desired effect, the incision cannot be truly limbal. As they are commonly performed, LRIs incorporate the outermost edge of the cornea, achieving the desired effect without compromising the corneal integrity. On the other hand, more central corneal relaxing incisions (CRIs) create the most powerful refractive change, but corneal integrity is sacrificed to some extent. The closer the incision is to the visual axis, the greater the effect, but smaller optical zones of 5 mm or less can produce severe glare and should be avoided.[1,2]

Nichamin LD.
Limbal Relaxing Incisions: A Practical Guide (pp 47-84).

Modern LRIs originated from the work of Dr. Stephen Hollis. I observed his technique of performing peripherally placed corneal incisions to correct residual astigmatism nearly 25 years ago. I incorporated his peripheral incisional technique to correct astigmatism at the time of cataract surgery and began using the term *limbal relaxing incisions*. Dr. Louis D. "Skip" Nichamin was also an early adopter of this technique and a pioneer of astigmatism correction.

LRIs have distinct advantages over CRIs. LRIs produce smoother, more homogenous corneal topographies and can be very effective in low to moderate astigmats (<3.00 diopters [D]). Because of their peripheral placement and longer length, LRIs tend to be more forgiving than CRIs, and the visual quality of the central cornea is preserved. The depth of the incisions, although important, is less critical than with CRIs. The more centrally placed corneal incisions may produce a "multifocal" effect,[3] are associated with a higher risk of overcorrection (even when treating small amounts of cylinder), and tend to be less predictable, particularly in patients with low amounts of astigmatism.

However, the effect of LRIs can be variable. The effect of LRIs is dependent on the patient's age, length of the incisions, depth of the incisions, and corneal thickness. These are all important considerations when developing the surgical plan.

Visualizing Astigmatism

Two-Dimensional Perspective

I visualize astigmatism in both 2 and 3 dimensions. When it comes to determining the placement and length of the incisions, I think of the cornea in clock hours. Because there are 360 degrees in a circle, each clock hour would equal 30 degrees, or 3 mm. Theoretically, a 3-mm or 30-degree incision would produce approximately 0.50 D of astigmatic correction.

Astigmatism in Three Dimensions

Many years ago, when I first tried to explain the concept of astigmatism to our technicians, I asked them to relate astigmatism to the 2 curves of a football—the "tip-to-tip" curve is the flat meridian, whereas the opposite curve that bisects the laces is the steep meridian. To explain with-the-rule and against-the-rule astigmatism, I used the visual of a football. With-the-rule astigmatism is demonstrated when a football is lying flat on the ground, and the flattest curve (tip to tip) is at 180 degrees (Figures 4-1 and 4-2). Imagining astigmatism in terms of shapes, rather than a flat, colored topography, makes terms such as *steep axis*, *flat axis*, and *coupling* more understandable and easier to visualize. This fundamental concept is critical for the entire team to understand.[4]

Continuing with the concept of the football, correcting astigmatism is a matter of altering the curves by "tightening the tip" or "loosening the laces" to create a more spherical shape. When applied to surgical procedures, we "loosen the laces" with astigmatic keratotomy to flatten a steep curve. We "tighten the tip" by suturing a relaxing incision. The tightening concept also applies to conductive keratoplasty, which can be used to correct small amounts of residual hyperopic astigmatism.

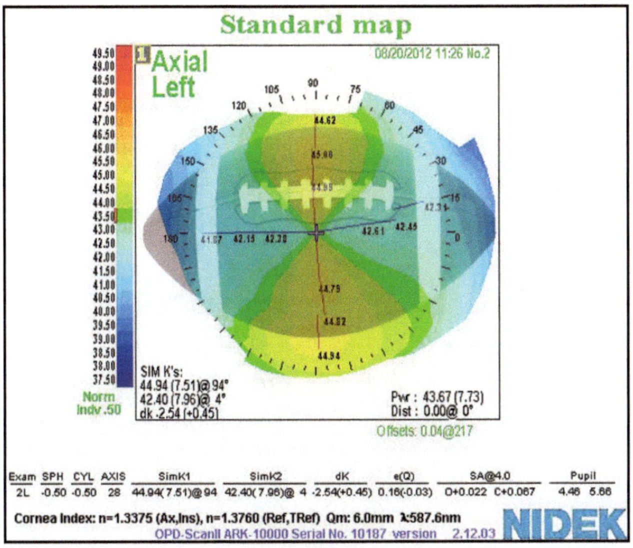

Figure 4-1. With-the-rule astigmatism is represented by a football lying on its side.

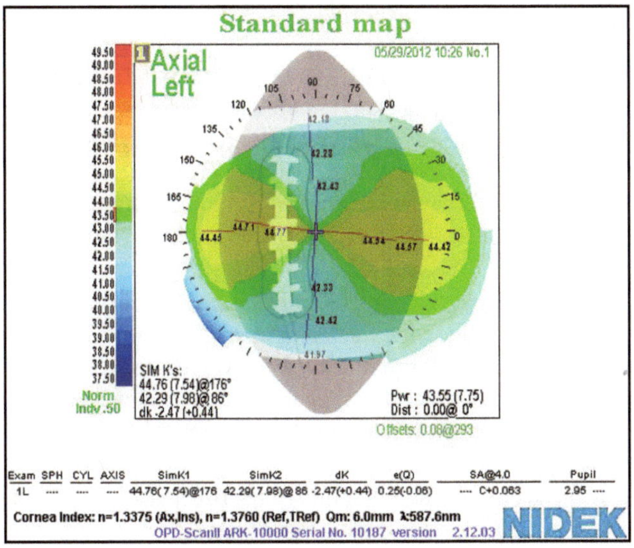

Figure 4-2. Against-the-rule astigmatism is represented by a football standing on end.

Technique for Astigmatism Correction in Conjunction With Cataract Surgery

Developing the Surgical Plan

When correcting astigmatism at the time of cataract surgery, our goal is to achieve a postoperative result of 0.50 D of astigmatism or less. When combined with the targeted spherical equivalent, the patient typically enjoys an excellent visual result. Some studies suggest that it can be beneficial to intentionally create a small amount of residual against-the-rule astigmatism to enhance near vision postoperatively.[5,6] However, those using presbyopic IOLs require a much lower tolerance for residual astigmatism (Dr. Kevin Miller, oral communication, 1998).

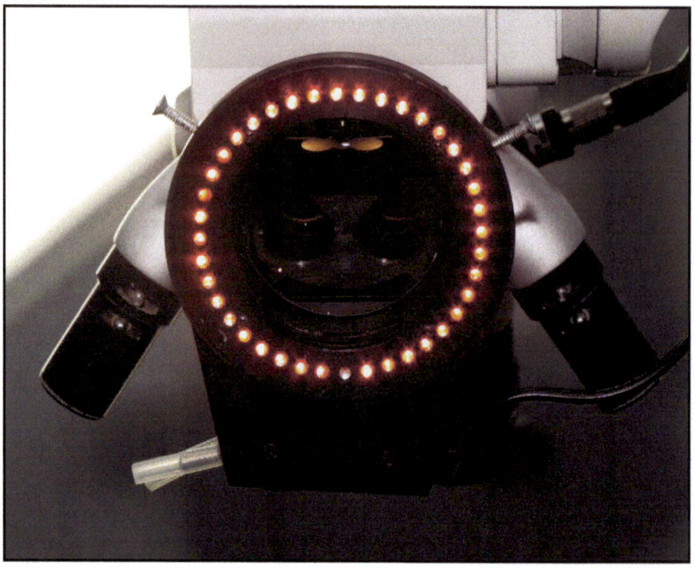

Figure 4-3. The Nevyas Operative Keratometer/360° Fixation Light (Varitronics Inc).

Understanding how to assess and assimilate the preoperative data is essential in developing the surgical plan. The refraction, topography, surgical keratometer (eg, Nevyas Operative Keratometer/360° Fixation Light; Varitronics Inc) (Figure 4-3), and pachymeter all provide critical data. The challenge is to determine which measurement is most relevant when the keratometric data do not agree. One study has shown the poor correlation among these measurements for assessing astigmatism, especially in patients with 2.00 D or less of astigmatism; this is where the "art" of astigmatism correction is applied.[7]

In the event of the phakic patient, the refractive cylinder is irrelevant because it can be either neutralized or exaggerated by lenticular cylinder. The lenticular component is removed by the cataract surgery and is not considered in the plan. We base our assessment, primarily with corneal topography, on the amount and the axis of precataract surgery astigmatism. However, we also rely heavily on intraoperative measurements from the surgical keratometer to assess the individual response to the placement and depth of the incision.

It is incumbent on the surgeon to assess the accuracy and reliability of the preoperative data. In our practice, the biometry team performs the corneal topography, keratometry, and pachymetry measurements. A standardized process reduces the variability from one staff member to another, and improves reproducibility. If there is doubt regarding a reasonable surgical plan, the astigmatism correction should be postponed until after cataract surgery and after there has been adequate time for wound healing. Secondary astigmatism correction can be performed at a later date.

In the event of patients who present with corneal pathology, such as Salzmann's nodular degeneration or Cogan's anterior basement membrane dystrophy, it may be necessary to perform a superficial keratectomy or phototherapeutic keratectomy to create a smooth corneal surface. When the cornea has re-epithelialized, a more accurate assessment and measurement of the cornea is possible, and it may then be incorporated into the cataract surgical plan.

Topography and Wavefront Analysis

Computerized topography and wavefront analysis are valuable tools in analyzing preoperative astigmatism. These modalities can identify corneal irregularities prior to performing a procedure so that the patient does not lose either best corrected vision or contrast sensitivity as a result of astigmatism correction. Topography and wavefront analysis can direct the treatment or the

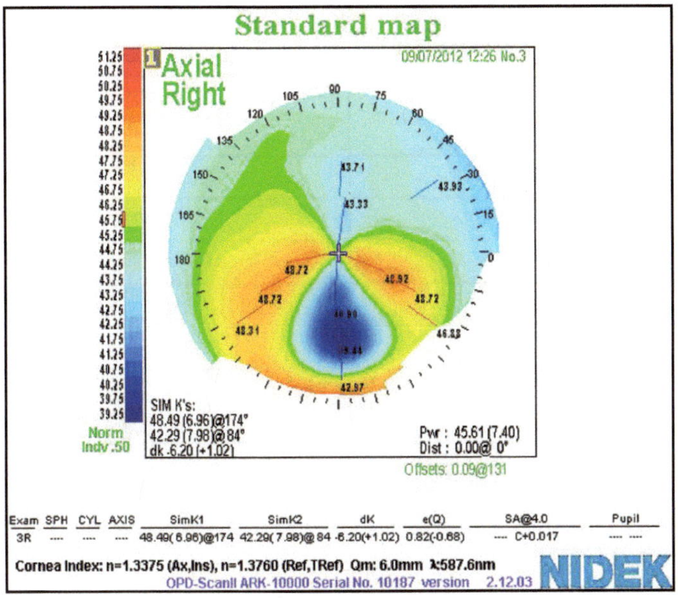

Figure 4-4. Topography map of pellucid marginal dystrophy; corneal relaxing incisions should be avoided.

observation of astigmatism by identifying irregular astigmatism, ectasia, forme fruste keratoconus, pellucid marginal dystrophy, and other higher-order aberrations[8] (Figure 4-4).

Higher-order aberrations are most commonly measured by the Shack-Hartmann aberrometer. This device measures the wavefront of the eye and compares it with an eye that has no aberrations. This aberration map is referred to as the eye's "optical fingerprint" because it is unique and unlike any other person's optical system.

Determining Incision Depth

During the early days of performing peripheral corneal incisions to correct astigmatism, we did not recognize the variability of the corneal thickness in our surgical plans and used preset blades. However, in recent years, measuring corneal thickness at the incision site has become an important part of surgical planning. Because the cornea varies in thickness from the center to periphery and in different meridia, it is important to measure pachymetry at the incision site. The blade depth is set to incise approximately 90% of the corneal thickness without perforation. Perforation is a risk, and in rare instances, corneal sutures are required. However, it is important to balance that risk while still achieving deep enough cuts to produce the desired effect.

Incision Size and Placement

All keratometric incisions flatten the cornea near the incision. The quadrant where the transverse or arcuate incision is placed will flatten, and flattening will also occur 180 degrees away from the incision. Keratometric incisions are always placed in the steep meridian.

I begin by drawing the plan for the incision placement on the patient's preoperative topography. I evaluate the pattern of astigmatism and place the relaxing incision according to the "bowtie," or the steep meridian on the corneal topography. If the astigmatism is regular, I make symmetrical incisions. However, if the astigmatism is asymmetrical, as in the case of keratoconus or form fruste keratoconus, manual LRIs should generally be avoided. The femtosecond laser does not yet have the ability to provide customized astigmatism correction; with the femtosecond laser, the incisions are automatically symmetrical or singular. When performing a manual LRI, it is possible to create

TABLE 4-1. GILLS LRI NOMOGRAM		
AMOUNT OF ASTIGMATISM	NUMBER OF INCISIONS	LENGTH OF INCISIONS
1 D	1	6 mm
2 D	2	6 mm
3 D	2	7 mm
4 D	2	8 mm
>4 D	2	10 mm
	CRIs based on correction desired over 4 D	2 mm for every D over 4 D at 8 mm OZ
LRI blade setting: 600 μm for most patients. CRI blade setting: 99% of pachymetry. (Exception: LRI blade setting of 500 μm for patients over 80 and for those with corneo-scleral thinning.)		

a longer incision on the steepest area (hemi-meridian) of the cornea, and a shorter incision in the relatively flatter half of the steep meridian.

If a patient has 2.00 to 3.00 D of astigmatism, I will usually make a pair of LRIs at the steep meridian, extending them up to 8 mm. The length and depth may be adjusted for age and corneal thickness.

Although the nomogram (Table 4-1) provides a starting point for the amount of astigmatism surgery to perform, the plan should be customized according to the topographic and surgical keratometer measurements. We use the Nevyas Operative Keratometer/360° Fixation Light to determine those measurements. Both the topography and the surgical keratometry are essential in planning for the individual variation in response. We start conservatively, using the surgical keratometer to gauge the effect of the procedure as it is performed. The ability to make adaptations to the surgical plan in real time is especially important with larger amounts of cylinder. By starting conservatively and closely following the impact of the procedure with the surgical keratometer, large over- and undercorrections can be avoided.

LRIs may be used to effect pre-existing astigmatism, in conjunction with the cataract incision. The type of cataract incision utilized generally depends on the type of lens used, as well as the location of the astigmatism. We perform a hinged incision, which is a variation of Langerman's 3-plane, self-sealing hinge incision for against-the-rule astigmatism eyes. When this type of incision is used, the initial groove, which is placed on the outer edge of the cornea, can be extended to incorporate the LRI. In these eyes, the impact of the cataract incision on the surgical plan does not need to be considered. For with-the-rule astigmatism, we perform scleral-limbal-corneal cataract incisions to minimize the amount of surgically induced corneal flattening. For those eyes, the LRI(s) is independent of the cataract incision.

Overcorrection

Overcorrection, which is rarer with LRIs than with CRIs, occasionally occurs. If I note an overcorrection in the early postoperative period, I prescribe sodium chloride drops 4 times a day. In rare instances, suturing the incision may be necessary if the overcorrection is large. I use the surgical keratometer to monitor the impact of the suture on the corneal shape. Both of these techniques work well; however, the best way to avoid overcorrections is to plan conservatively for a slight undercorrection. It is much simpler to enhance an undercorrection postoperatively than to manage an overcorrection. In addition, patients seem to be more tolerant of a slight undercorrection rather than a slight overcorrection.

Incorporating the Principle of Coupling in the Surgical Plan

Coupling is a term that describes the change in corneal power at the incision site compared with the change in corneal power 90 degrees away. The coupling ratio is the amount of flattening produced by an incision relative to the flattening or steepening 90 degrees away. Incisions, such as with radial keratotomy, produce a coupling ratio of 1:1, which is an equal amount of flattening at the incision site and 90 degrees away. This flattening produces a hyperopic shift, whereas steepening produces a myopic shift. Therefore, the term *maximum coupling* denotes a low coupling ratio.

It is possible for 2 procedures to correct the same amount of astigmatism but produce a different coupling ratio. For example, a single, long LRI produces a greater hyperopic shift (or higher coupling ratio) than 2 shorter CRIs (which produce a low coupling ratio). Shorter incisions require more central placement and should be within a 15-degree arc. When shorter incisions are used, there is a lower coupling ratio and thus less impact on the postoperative spherical equivalent.

Impact of Coupling on Primary and Secondary Astigmatic Keratotomy

Understanding the coupling ratio of a given astigmatic procedure is important to take into consideration when selecting the IOL power. For example, if a patient has 1.00 D of asymmetrical astigmatism, the plan may be to perform a single, 6-mm LRI. In this instance, because a hyperopic shift is anticipated as a result of a high coupling ratio (due to the use of a single relaxing incision), it is important to add power to the IOL to achieve the desired spherical equivalent.

With secondary astigmatism correction, this concept is particularly important because the impact of the coupling ratio is solely dependent on the astigmatic incisions and cannot be neutralized by the IOL. With secondary relaxing incisions, the decision to use limbal or corneal incisions should be based on whether the patient has a hyperopic, myopic, or neutral spheroequivalent and the desired outcome.[9] Our outcomes analysis show that approximately half of the patients who receive 2 LRIs of approximately 6 mm in length will experience approximately 0.50 D of hyperopic shift. Although this does not occur in 100% of eyes, it is still better to add 0.50 D of power to the IOL than for the patient to have the undesirable outcome of hyperopia.

In the instance of a patient with residual secondary astigmatism and a hyperopic spherical equivalent, a low coupling ratio (myopic shift) is the desired effect. However, producing a low coupling ratio is more difficult, but it is possible. This can be accomplished if the incisions are kept within a 15-degree arc, are placed in the 7- to 9-mm optical zone, and more than one pair is performed to produce the desired correction. Such incisions are short and stepped. The number of incisions used may be placed as multiple pairs. Using the technique of using short, stepped corneal incisions, rather than longer, limbal incisions, minimizes the hyperopic shift on the spherical equivalent. The coupling effect is maximized when there is greater steepening 90 degrees away from where the incision is made. In this instance, a coupling ratio of nearly 1:1 can be achieved.

Limbal Relaxing Incisions Versus Toric Intraocular Lens Implantation

Although it is possible to correct moderate to higher amounts of astigmatism with astigmatic keratotomy, the advent and recent advances in toric IOLs presents a viable and, in some cases, preferable alternative. The silicone plate design of the STAAR Surgical Company's toric IOL caused early rotation that had to be managed prior to capsular fusion. Although the issue of rotation could be managed fairly easily, it was not ideal. With the availability of the AcrySof toric IOL (Alcon Surgical) in the United States, with powers ranging from 1.50 to 6.00 D thereby yielding correction from 1.00 to 4.00 D, our ability to manage astigmatism has been further expanded. Additional toric implants are available internationally, including multifocal designs.

Our experience with the aspheric AcrySof toric lens has produced excellent optical results, and its acrylic polymer material has an adhesive nature that minimizes rotation within the capsular bag.[10,11] Although rotation is less of an issue compared with earlier silicone plate–haptic designs, it has been known to occur in high myopia patients. In these rare cases, we wait until the capsule has begun to contract, and then we rotate the lens to the proper axis. These lenses are also ideal for younger patients, where the corneal response to astigmatic keratotomy may be less predictable.

Despite the potential advantages of toric implants, they are not indicated for every patient. These IOLs are optimal for patients with regular, symmetrical, and bowtie astigmatism, but they could actually induce astigmatism in patients with either irregular astigmatism or asymmetrical bowtie corneal topographic patterns. We generally use LRIs for low amounts of astigmatism and incorporate the use of toric IOLs for moderate-to-high levels. In addition, the cost of toric lenses is significantly higher than LRIs and is a consideration for some patients, particularly those with low-to-moderate astigmatism.

For patients who undergo cataract surgery with toric IOL implantation, LRI remains an excellent means to enhance the result following surgery. This is particularly true for those patients with higher amounts of astigmatism.

Astigmatism Management With Femtosecond Laser and Toric Intraocular Lens Implantation

Pit Gills, MD

The introduction of femtosecond laser technology to correct astigmatism holds promise for adding a new level of accuracy to the use of corneal and LRIs (see Chapter 7). I have found one of the greatest attributes of the femtosecond laser is its ability to create arcuate incisions. These incisions are more corneal than (intra-) limbal, although the surgeon has complete control over the optical zone, length, and depth of the incision. When performing a relaxing incision manually, the depth of the incision may vary depending on the applied pressure and the blade angle induced by the surgeon. Femtosecond technology incorporates real-time optical coherence tomography. This provides the surgeon with precise corneal thickness measurements at the exact location of the arcuate incision. This level of accuracy allows one to maximize the depth of the arcuate incision while lowering the risk of perforation.

The femtosecond arcuate incision can be performed alone or in combination with toric IOL implantation. The benefit of combining arcuate incisions created by the femtosecond laser with a toric implant is twofold. First, the arcuate incisions serve as excellent markers to confirm proper alignment of the toric IOL while in the operating room. Although we still mark the cornea and use the surgical keratometer intraoperatively, the level of control and precision of incision placement results in a significantly lower number of lens repositioning procedures.

Second, when using the femtosecond laser to create the arcuate incision, we have the option to create an internal (intrastromal) CRI, while leaving the epithelium sealed. By leaving the epithelium intact, it results in an incision that effectively produces little effect on corneal astigmatism. This allows us to "fine tune" the patient's postoperative result by breaking the epithelial seal and then titrating toward the intended correction.

Despite the effort to obtain accurate preoperative measurements, the theoretical surgical plan does not always match the empirical data of the surgical outcome. In this regard, I find the use of titrating laser incisions in combination with toric implants to be very helpful. For example, I use the femtosecond laser to create a pair of 15-degree incisions in the steep meridian. I use those incisions as the marks to align the hash marks of the toric lens. In an instance where the toric power was conservative and the patient had residual astigmatism in the same axis, one or both of the corneal incisions can subsequently be opened to increase the amount of correction. I do this at the slit lamp with a drop of proparacaine ophthalmic, using a Slade femtosecond spatula (Asico, LLC). Depending on the postoperative refraction and topography, the extent of this postoperative adjustment can be titrated. Although the impact of a 15-degree arcuate incision is small, the ability to fine tune the patient's postoperative result has proven to be a valuable tool.

Biaspheric Lenses

The use of biaspheric lenses has provided a significant advancement in improving our patients' quality of vision.[12] The strategy of the biaspheric design is to reduce spherical aberration by controlling paraxial light rays, as they intersect at the paraxial focal point instead of in front of or behind it. This effect is the opposite of that which may occur with the use of multifocal IOLs, which tend to amplify corneal aberrations and thus increase undesirable dysphotopsia and degrade optical quality. Biaspheric lenses, on the other hand, minimize these aberrations. For patients with peripheral corneal astigmatism, the effect of LRIs can be enhanced because of the optical properties of the lenses. This is a particularly important consideration in patients with previous radial keratotomy, pterygia, and other conditions that induce irregular astigmatism, where splitting of light must be avoided.

In short, there is no "one size fits all" approach to correcting astigmatism. Each patient's individual needs, expectations, topography analysis, refractive error, and IOL selection must be considered to develop a customized surgical plan. In addition, the surgeon must remain nimble and ready during the procedure to make adjustments to the plan based on the individual response from the surgical keratometer. Finally, close postoperative follow-up, with the cooperation of an optometric team to evaluate the refractive error, is required.

Astigmatism Pearls

- *Creating the plan.* Use your nomogram of choice as a starting point rather than an absolute guide. Consider the amount and orientation of the cylinder when developing the surgical plan.
- *Toric IOL implantation vs LRIs.* Avoid disruption of the corneal surface for patients with Fuchs' dystrophy or surface issues, such as anterior basement membrane or Cogan's dystrophy. Because these patients are usually better candidates for toric IOL implantation, opt for a toric lens to avoid disruption of the corneal surface.
- *Treat irregular astigmatism uniquely.* Set expectations carefully, explaining and documenting the limitations of correcting irregular astigmatism. Because toric lenses cannot completely

correct irregular astigmatism, these patients should expect improvement, not perfection. When selecting the cylinder power of a toric IOL, lean toward undercorrection rather than overcorrection.

- *Standardize your measurement process.* Train specific staff to perform preoperative measurements. Even with automated equipment, such as topography and the IOLMaster biometer (Carl Zeiss Meditec Inc), it is beneficial to identify key staff to perform measurements for better continuity and accuracy.
- *Maximize the benefits of the femtosecond laser.* When performing astigmatism correction with the femtosecond laser, along with toric IOL implantation, incorporate a pair of arcuate incisions that could be used to titrate the amount of astigmatism postoperatively. These incisions have the added benefit of markers for the toric IOL alignment.

References

1. Lavery G. Clinical results of trapezoidal astigmatic keratotomy. *J Refract Surg.* 1985;1:70-74.
2. Gills JP, Fenzl RE. Analysis of astigmatic keratotomy with a 5.0 mm optical clear zone. *Am J Ophthalmol.* 1996;121(6):731-732.
3. Gills JP. Corneal relaxing incisions, multifocal corneas, and "omnimetropia." In: Gills JP, Sanders DR, Thornton SP, Martin, RG, Gayton JL, Holladay JT, eds. *Corneal Topography: The State of the Art.* Thorofare, NJ: SLACK Incorporated; 1995:225-239.
4. Gills JP. Football mnemonic for correction of preoperative astigmatism. *J Am Introcul Implant Soc.* 1983;9(1):57.
5. Verzella F, Calossi A. Multifocal effect of against-the-rule myopic astigmatism in pseudophakic eyes. *J Refract Corneal Surg.* 1993;9(1):58-61.
6. Sawusch M, Guyton D. Optimal astigmatism to enhance depth of focus after cataract surgery. *Ophthalmology.* 1991;98(7):1025-1029.
7. Wallace RB. On-axis cataract incisions: where is the axis? 1995 ASCRS Symposium of Cataract, IOL and Refractive Surgery "Best Papers of Sessions." 1995;67-72.
8. Saad A, Gatinel D. Evaluation of total and corneal wavefront high order aberrations for the detection of forme fruste keratoconus. *Invest Ophthalmol Vis Sci.* 2012 17;53(6):2978-2992.
9. Gills JP, Rowsey JJ. Managing coupling in secondary astigmatic keratotomy. *Int Ophthalmol Clin.* 2003;43(3):29-41.
10. Kershner RM. Retinal image contrast and functional visual performance with aspheric, silicone, and acrylic intraocular lenses. *J Cataract Refract Surg.* 2003;29(9):1684-1694.
11. Trueb PR, Albach C, Montes-Milco R, Ferrer-Blasco T. Visual acuity and contrast sensitivity in eyes implanted with aspheric and spherical intraocular lenses. *Ophthalmology.* 2009;116(5):890-895.
12. Brown DC, Gills JP III, Trattler WB, Newsom TH, Weinstock RJ, Sanders DR. Prospective multicenter trial assessing effectiveness, refractive predictability and safety of a new aberration free, bi-aspheric intraocular lens. *Cont Lens Anterior Eye.* 2011;34(4):188-192.

Section 2: How I Perform Limbal Relaxing Incisions

Richard S. Hoffman, MD

Limbal relaxing incision (LRI) is one of the simplest and most useful techniques for enhancing the results from cataract and refractive lens exchange surgery. The success of implementing LRIs into your surgical armamentarium may be maximized with attention to a thorough preoperative assessment, including preoperative testing and patient counseling, in addition to systematically performing the technique and addressing postoperative care. My approach for offering and implementing LRIs may have slightly different nuances than other surgeons. However, the beauty of LRIs lies in their success, despite different approaches and possible inaccuracies in technique. Each surgeon has reasons and pearls for performing LRIs using their particular method, and knowledge can always be gained by understanding their unique approach. My current method for offering and performing LRIs is outlined in this section.

Preoperative Assessment

Before I step into the room to evaluate a patient who may require cataract surgery, the ophthalmic technicians will have performed automated keratometry measurements, in addition to a manifest refraction. In addition to these, measurements, I recently instituted the use of a no-charge computerized corneal topographic map (CCT). Having this information available to me before I recommend a particular intraocular lens (IOL) model or the use of LRIs has been extremely useful for talking intelligently with the patient and for improving office efficiency by avoiding the need to change the decision regarding the surgical approach after informed consent has been given. The use of automated keratometry and screening CCTs has stemmed from many instances in which a patient was found to have large amounts of refractive cylinder that was lenticular in nature rather than corneal, which was discovered only after biometry was performed for IOL calculations. In addition, some patients have been found to have small amounts of refractive cylinder and were later found to have large amounts of corneal astigmatism that would benefit from LRIs or toric IOL implantation. Perhaps there is no greater way to shake a patient's confidence in your skills or the skills of your technicians than by approaching him or her after the informed consent has been discussed and then changing the surgical plan due to newly discovered corneal astigmatism, or the lack of corneal astigmatism, due to significant refractive cylinder.

Although many surgeons defer the discussion of financial issues to their surgical coordinator or scheduler, I prefer to inform the patient of the costs of LRIs, toric IOLs, and presbyopia-correcting IOLs before the informed consent process. In my practice, cost seems to be a major factor in which modality, if any, a patient will choose. If I mention the cost of an LRI to a patient and explain that his or her insurance does not cover this service, and if the patient appears to balk at the relatively low expense, I can then save myself a lot of time by not going through the explanation of the procedure. I can also avoid offering the more expensive alternative of toric IOL implantation. Every patient with clinically significant astigmatism is made aware of his or her options, including LRIs, toric IOLs, and especially the option of correcting the astigmatism with spectacles postoperatively.

The greatest need for LRIs is in patients who have corneal astigmatism and who opt for a presbyopia-correcting IOL implantation. In the United States there is currently no toric multifocal IOL available for patients. Multifocal and accommodative IOLs will usually not function at an acceptable level if greater than 0.75 diopters (D) of astigmatism is present. This leaves the surgeon who offers patients presbyopia-correcting IOLs within the United States, the responsibility of addressing pre-existing astigmatism with either LRIs or excimer laser corneal refractive surgery. When patients present with large amounts of corneal astigmatism (usually greater than 2.00 to 2.50 D), I inform them of the risks or likelihood of residual astigmatism that might deliver suboptimum visual quality in the presence of such premium IOLs. I also inform them of the options for addressing the residual astigmatism with laser in situ keratomileusis (LASIK) or photorefractive keratectomy (PRK), and I also inform them of the additional costs for excimer laser refractive enhancements.

All patients undergoing LRIs or toric IOLs are advised of the possible need for enhancements, toric IOL repositioning, and the general risks for IOL surgery. For patients who are undergoing LRIs in combination with monofocal IOL implantation, I inform them that I am going to attempt to reduce, but not necessarily eliminate, their astigmatism. In this way, patients will (hopefully) not return with complaint of 0.50 D of residual cylinder.

As part of our preoperative testing, we perform biometry for axial length, in addition to automated keratometry and CCT. Pachymetry measurements are taken at the steep axis just

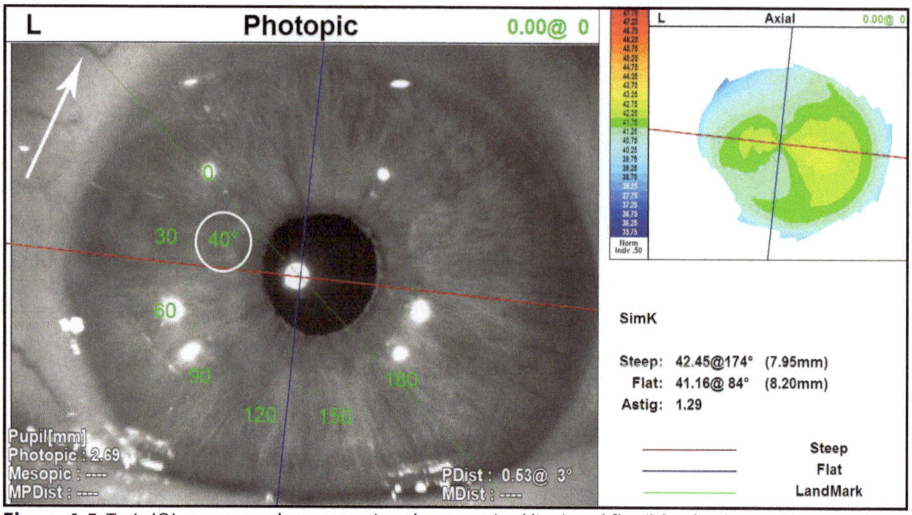

Figure 4-5. Toric IOL summary demonstrating the steep (red line) and flat (blue line) meridians overlying the eye image. The green axis reticule has been rotated to a prominent L- shaped vessel (white arrow). The measured angle is 40 degrees from the sclera vessel to the steep meridian (white circle).

inside the limbus, corresponding to the locations of both matching LRIs. These measurements are placed within our electronic medical record and also are recorded on the printed CCT map corresponding to the location of the steep axis. In addition, the 90% depth is calculated and recorded in the electronic medical record and attached to the surgical plan that is displayed within the operating suite.

We have recently acquired a new combined CCT/wavefront analyzer from NIDEK Inc—the OPD-Scan III. This device has a feature termed the *Toric IOL Summary*. Basically, at the time the eye is imaged, a photograph is taken that has the steep and flat axis displayed overlying the cornea. A green reticule can then be easily manipulated to correspond to an iris landmark or prominent scleral vessel. The image will then display the number of degrees from that landmark to the steep axis (Figure 4-5). The information is then stored, and, during surgery, the image can be displayed and the surgeon can then use an LRI marker that is set to the number of degrees from the landmark. This summary allows the ability to accurately determine the steep axis intraoperatively without having to mark the vertical or horizontal meridians with the patient sitting up. Regardless of the amount of cyclotorsion in the supine position, the steep axis will always be at the same measured increment from the surface landmark. I have found this system to be extremely accurate for lining up toric IOLs and LRIs, and, on several occasions, it appeared to be more accurate than marking the 12- and 6-o'clock meridia with a marking pen. The system does require a prominent surface landmark, which is not always present, thus, traditional limbal marking will still be required in many patients.

If irregular or asymmetric astigmatism is discovered on the CCT, the surgeon will need to decide if the treatment is wise in general and/or if the nomograms will need to be adjusted. For frank irregular astigmatism due to corneal ectasia or forme fruste keratoconus, I believe LRIs should be avoided due to their inconsistent response. Corneal relaxing incisions at a 7- or 8-mm optical zone are definitely contraindicated. When the astigmatism is asymmetric and minimally skewed, I believe LRIs can be performed with good success. The nomogram for these eyes is adjusted somewhat in that one LRI would be made longer with a greater angle of arc corresponding to the greater cylinder power at that limbal location. In the same way, the other side might be adjusted down to a smaller angle that corresponds to the smaller angle of steepness. This adjustment of the nomogram is more art than science, but it basically follows the relative contribution of each end of the cylinder bowtie to the overall cylinder.

The Procedure

A host of different ways of determining the steep meridian of astigmatism is available, including surface landmarks, microscope-mounted keratoscopes, hand-held keratoscopes, and preoperative or intraoperative limbal marking. The simplest method of marking the steep axis to use as axis reference points is to mark the limbus with a fine gentian violet marking pen at either the 12- and 6-o'clock meridians or the 3- and 9-o'clock meridians. There are special devices available for insuring that these reference marks are accurately placed, including markers with carpenter's bubble levels and gravity weights; however, I prefer to manually place a mark at 12- and 6-o'clock meridians by eye. The most essential point when making these reference marks is to ensure that the patient is sitting upright and looking straight ahead. Marking in the supine position is prohibited due to the confounding effects of cyclotorsion. These reference marks are usually made by one of our technicians in the "holding area," and then they are enhanced on the operating table if necessary using a Sinskey hook (Katena Products) stained with additional dye.

The surgical plan is determined preoperatively and is calculated using a traditional Nichamin nomogram with the diamond knife set to 90% of the preoperative pachymetric measurement. My standard cataract technique utilizes 2 1.0-mm bimanual incisions at the temporal oblique meridia, followed by a 2.2-mm temporal clear corneal incision for IOL insertion, all being beveled and single-plane in design. If one of the LRI incisions is in the same axis as the bimanual incision, I will usually rotate the bimanual incision to a location outside the placement of the LRI. For the coaxial surgeon, the paracentesis should be rotated to a different meridian if the LRI is in the same oblique location. This involves a few seconds of mentally locating the LRIs on the eye prior to placing the paracentesis or microincisions. If the steep axis is at 180 degrees, the LRIs will be placed at the beginning of the procedure, and the temporal clear corneal cataract incision will be placed at the 50% depth within the temporal LRI. For large temporal LRIs, some surgeons will make the temporal LRI of only 30 degrees, so that the wound is not distorted during phacoemulsification and then widen the LRI following it. I personally have found that phacoemulsification through a 2.2-mm incision made within a large 60-degree LRI is not problematic and saves the step of having to widen the LRI.

Ordinarily, I prefer to make my LRIs after phacoemulsification is performed (bimanually) but before IOL implantation for several reasons. First, there is a small risk of perforation of the LRI, despite accurate pachymetric measurements. Before I was performing pachymetry preoperatively, I did note several instances of perforated LRIs in eyes that had a limbal thickness of less than the standard 600 µm, which was routinely used for diamond knife settings. A perforated LRI requires suturing, and, even in the best of hands, balanced salt solution will continuously squirt out of these perforated incisions, making the surgery more challenging. A perforation at the end of the procedure avoids this mess. Second, there is the remote possibility of the occurrence of intraoperative complications, requiring widening of the clear corneal incision or scleral fixation of IOLs. These alterations in the surgical plan will sabotage the astigmatic treatments and may actually worsen the cylinder, depending on the complication, treatment, and location of the original LRIs. The rational for placing the LRIs before IOL placement stems from the potential for retinal toxicity if the microscope is left focusing its strong coherent light beam through an emmetropic IOL for any prolonged period of time. LRIs can usually be made in less than 1 minute; however, in the novice's hand or in the presence of unforeseen delays, retinal phototoxicity is a real danger that can be avoided if the IOL is placed after all other adjunctive procedures have been performed.

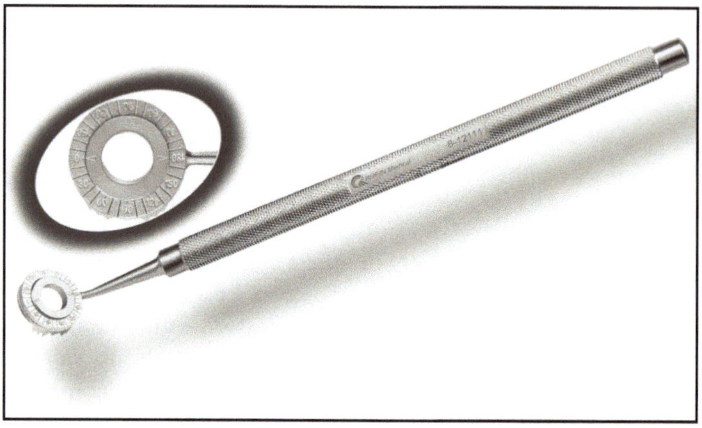

Figure 4-6. Dell astigmatism marker (Rhein Medical Ophthalmic Surgical Instruments, #8-12111). (Reprinted with permission from Rhein Medical Inc.)

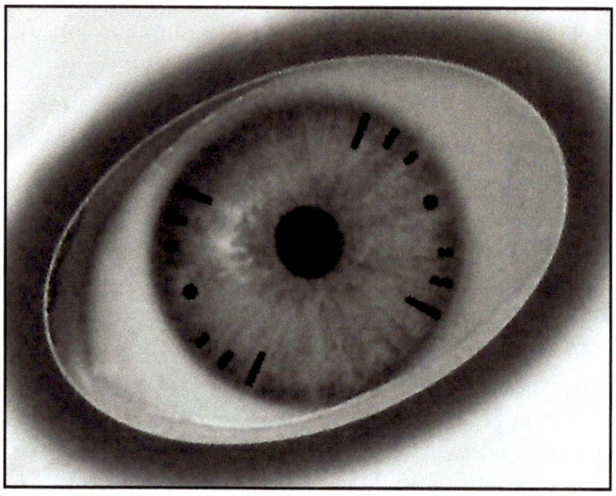

Figure 4-7. Marking stamp pattern of the Dell astigmatism marker. The distance from the first small radial marks on either side of the round dot corresponds to 40 degrees. The distance from the next two radial marks is 60 degrees. The distance from the outer longer radial marks to each other is 80 degrees.

Technique

After cortical clean-up, a cohesive viscoelastic is placed within the capsular bag and the anterior chamber to pressurize the eye to 20 to 30 mm Hg. ASICO LLC has created a special LRI marker for me that will imprint radial marks corresponding to 40-, 60-, and 80-degree LRIs on a rotating bezel that can be set to the steep meridian. In addition, the marker has tines at the 90- and 270-degree meridians. These marks will form on the conjunctiva just outside of the corneal limbus and are used to confirm that the marker was lined up with the preplaced 12-o'clock orientation marks. Rhein Medical Ophthalmic Surgical Instruments has created a similar marker—the Dell Astigmatism Marker (8-12111) (Figures 4-6 and 4-7).

The limbus corresponding to where the LRIs will be placed is dried with a Merocel sponge (Beaver Visitec). The LRI marker is then set to the steep meridian and pressed against a gentian violet pad. The axis of the marker is double-checked under the microscope because of the possibility of bezel rotation after contact with the dye pad. The marker is then pressed against the cornea, lining the 90- and 270-degree meridia of the marker with the 12- and 6-o'clock conjunctival reference marks. Quickly removing the marker will usually guarantee that sharp radial marks have been placed. If needed, the marks corresponding to the planned LRI arcs can be augmented with a Sinskey hook dipped in the dye. A small quantity of viscoelastic is then placed at the limbus overlying the radial marks to help reduce epithelial tearing from the diamond LRI knife.

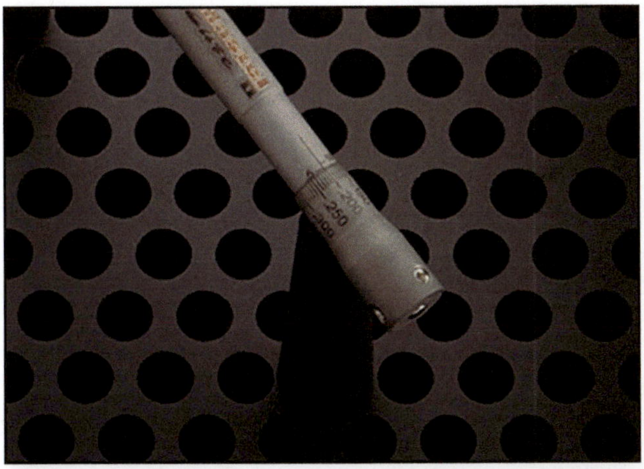

Figure 4-8. Fully adjustable micrometer on the Mastel Elite II diamond knife (Mastel Precision Ophthalmic Surgical Instruments Inc). (Reprinted with permission from Mastel Precision.)

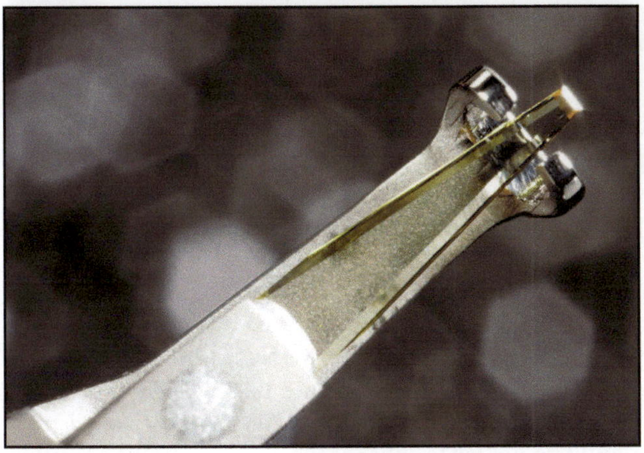

Figure 4-9. C-shaped footplate on the Mastel Elite II diamond knife (Mastel Precision Ophthalmic Surgical Instruments Inc). (Reprinted with permission from Mastel Precision.)

Diamond knives that are made for LRIs come in various designs and assortments, including fixed-depth knives, adjustable knives, and knives with different footplate designs. I believe that knives with one depth setting should be avoided, and knives with 3 depth settings also have their limitations. When I first started performing LRIs, I used a knife that was preset at 600 µm. Although this worked well for the majority of cases, I subsequently found that many eyes had a limbal thickness that was much greater than 600 µm, and a few had very thin limbal thickness less than 600 µm. I believe that many of my cases of gross undercorrections or regressions were secondary to utilizing a 600-µm blade in a cornea that may have had a thickness between 750 and 800 µm at the limbus. Obviously, the thinner corneas were the ones with perforations. It is because of these nuances that I now use a diamond knife with an adjustable micrometer so that the blade can be consistently set to 90% depth. My current blade of preference is the Mastel Elite II (Mastel Precision Ophthalmic Surgical Instruments Inc) (Figure 4-8), with a C-shaped guarded footplate (Figure 4-9).

During the procedure, the globe is fixated with a Fine-Thornton ring (Mastel Precision Ophthalmic Surgical Instruments Inc) (Figure 4-10), and the blade enters the cornea perpendicular to the surface, 1 mm inside of the limbus. In my opinion, placing the LRI in the white tissue of the limbus results in undercorrection due to excessive healing, so I prefer to err on placing the incisions in clear cornea 1 mm anterior to the limbus. Although right-handed surgeons can use the right hand to make both incisions, I prefer to use an ambidextrous approach, especially when sitting temporally and making incisions at the superior and inferior limbus. Care should be made

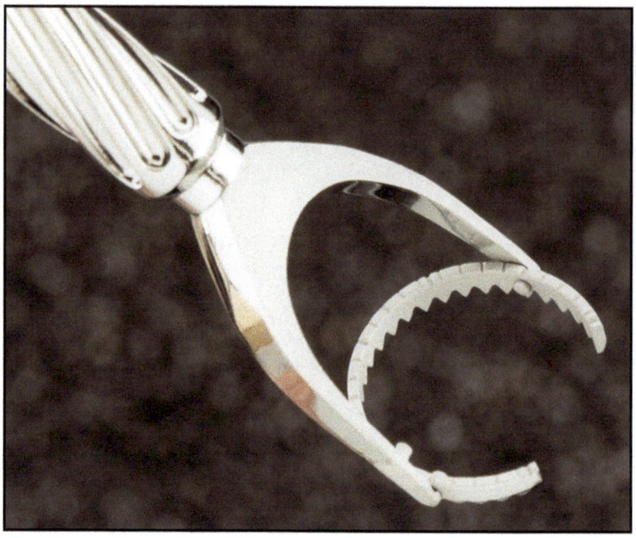

Figure 4-10. Fine-Thornton fixation ring (Mastel Precision Ophthalmic Surgical Instruments Inc). (Reprinted with permission from Mastel Precision.)

to ensure that the footplate remains flush with the globe throughout the extent of the incision and that the blade is not torqued. This is especially important if "single ski" straight footplates are used, as the footplate can enter into the LRI, creating a deeper incision if the blade is torqued. After the incisions have been made to the appropriate length, the depth should be checked and the incisions should be irrigated with balanced salt solution from a 30-gauge cannula.

Although various tools can be used to assess the effect from the LRIs, including hand-held and operating microscope–mounted keratoscopes and wavefront analyzers, I have found these devices to be somewhat unreliable immediately after creating the incisions. This is especially true if a temporal clear corneal incision was made for phacoemulsification because this incision is stretched and hydrated to varying degrees during the cataract extraction. Thus, for the most part, I trust my measurements and the nomograms, and I do not try to enhance the incisions on the operating table.

Since performing pachymetry preoperatively, I believe I have not had a perforation during an LRI. If a perforation is created, the blade progression should be stopped immediately at the first sign of viscoelastic egress. Multiple radial 10-0 nylon sutures with light tension should be placed, and antibiotic coverage should be continued for 1 to 2 weeks. Sutures can be removed 4 to 6 weeks following surgery. Interestingly, I have found that the full effect from the LRIs can still be appreciated when all sutures have been removed if the full LRI arc was created. Reassuring patients to this fact can help alleviate the anxiety that may be produced from the sutures-in astigmatism that is created from the wound closure.

Postoperative Care

Following cataract surgery with LRIs, standard postoperative medications are utilized. Antibiotics are used 4 times a day for 1 week, nonsteroidal medications for 2 weeks, and topical steroids 3 to 4 times a day for 1 month. If unacceptable cylinder remains following surgery, I will usually wait at least 1 month before performing an enhancement. Enhancements can be created by either deepening the original LRIs or increasing the arc length. If pachymetry was performed preoperatively and the diamond knife was set accurately to 90% depth, then redeepening will usually not be effective. LRI lengthening is perhaps the best means of increasing the astigmatic effect and can be easily performed at the slit lamp. Overcorrections with cylinder axis shifting of 90 degrees are extremely rare.

The slit-lamp enhancements are performed with topical proparacaine. Pachymetry is repeated at the steep meridian, and the LRI marker is set to the steep axis. Marking of the 12-o'clock axis is not necessary because the patient will be in the upright position, eliminating any cyclotorsion. With a lid speculum in place and the patient's head in the slit lamp, the LRI marker is pressed against a gentian violet pad and pressed onto the eye surface after the correct axis on the marker is confirmed. The LRI blade is set to 90-degrees depth. The previous LRIs are easily opened with a sterile Sinskey hook, and the incisions are lengthened 5 to 10 degrees on either side of the incision, depending on the amount of undercorrection. No fixation of the globe is needed with a cooperative patient. In instances where there is a significant error in the postoperative spherical equivalent in addition to residual cylinder, I will perform PRK. LASIK is usually avoided due to the risks of epithelial ingrowth from a keratectomy flap cutting through the previous LRI incisions.

In the rare instance where the LRIs may have been placed in the wrong axis, wait 1 month and then repeat the LRIs as if the eye was virgin. Essentially, the new plan is based on the new astigmatism and the new axis. The cylinder correction will usually behave as if the LRIs were done for the first time.

Most importantly, treat the patient and not the refractive error. If a patient has 1.00 D of residual astigmatism and is happy, leave him or her alone. If the patient has 20/30 vision and happy, leave him or her alone. Do not mess with 20/happy. The opposite may be said for the 20/20 unhappy patient. A patient with a multifocal IOL, 20/20 vision, and 0.50 D of residual cylinder might seem like a poor candidate for enhancement, but sometimes just making the effort to improve his or her quality of vision with either a PRK or LRI enhancement can turn the patient from 20/20 unhappy to 20/happy.

Final Comments

I believe that the LRI is one of the simplest and most useful tools in the ophthalmologist's armamentarium, and I am still amazed at how many surgeons register for LRI courses at our national meetings and are not trained in this technique. For surgeons practicing within the United States who plan on utilizing multifocal IOLs, the ability to perform LRIs is indispensable. LRIs are also a wonderful means of patient advertising, as these individuals tend to be satisfied with their uncorrected vision and are very likely to rave about their vision to their friends and neighbors.

LRIs are easy to master with a short learning curve. The incisions are extremely forgiving with overcorrections, and significant undercorrections are rare when they are properly performed. The equipment needed to perform LRIs is relatively inexpensive, and the costs can be quickly recouped because the procedure is not covered by insurance or Medicare, and most patients are willing to pay the small out-of-pocket expense to enhance their refractive result. In fact, in my practice, LRIs will actually save patients money, as they are less expensive to perform relative to the cost of toric IOLs. LRIs are simple, fast, effective, and safe.

Key Points

- Perform keratometry before discussing LRIs.
- Perform computerized corneal topography to confirm astigmatism and rule out ectatic disorders.
- Place limbal reference marks with the patient sitting upright and looking straight ahead at a fixation target.

- If preoperative astigmatism is at 180 degrees, place the LRIs at the beginning of the procedure and place the clear corneal cataract incision within the temporal incision. For all other meridians, perform the LRIs after phacoemulsification but before IOL implantation.
- Placing a small quantity of viscoelastic over the epithelium in the region of the LRI may reduce the likelihood for epithelial tearing.
- LRI enhancements can be performed 1 month following the initial surgery at the slit lamp in most patients by re-marking and lengthening the original incisions.

Section 3: Astigmatism Correction With Peripheral Corneal Relaxing Incision

Douglas D. Koch, MD and Christian C. Hester, MD

In preparation for a peripheral corneal relaxing incision (PCRI), we obtain corneal measurements with at least 2 devices, one of which is a corneal topographer. Astigmatism can be quantified by manual or automated keratometry (eg, IOLMaster [Carl Zeiss Meditec Inc] or LENSTAR [Haag-Streit USA]). In our practice, we use corneal topography and a Scheimpflug analyzer to (1) ensure that astigmatism is regular, (2) rule out ectatic disorders, and (3) assess peripheral corneal thickness. We require that agreement between device measurements is within 0.50 diopters (D) and 10 degrees.

Marking the Cornea

Accurate landmarks are critical for the successful correction of astigmatism with PCRIs. Preoperatively, the corneal and conjunctival epithelia should be marked at the 90- or 180-degree meridian. Because the average eye will cyclotort by at least 4 degrees when the patient moves from an upright to a supine position, the markings should be made while the patient is in an upright position. For each degree of rotation, the effect of the PCRI is lessened by 3.33%.[1] When using a slit lamp, align a thin beam through the center of the pupil at the desired semi-meridian. Next, score the corneal epithelium with a Sinskey hook (Eye Supply USA) stained with gentian violet dye. If the epithelium is not penetrated with the Sinskey hook, the mark will disappear (Figure 4-11). When a slit lamp is not available, have the patient sit in an upright position and fixate on an object straight ahead with the operative eye. With a fine tip marking pen, mark the corneal and conjunctival epithelia at the 90- or 180-degree meridian (Figure 4-12).

After making the marks, evaluate their location. It is important to note the position of the marks in case they are not perfectly placed. Make a drawing indicating the precise location of the marks relative to the intended site and take this drawing to the operating room. Intraoperatively, the premarked semi-meridians serve as a reference point for the astigmatic marker to identify and mark the desired steep meridian (Figure 4-13). Alternatively, one can use one of several commercially available markers to mark the steep semi-meridians directly, obviating the need for marking them intraoperatively.

Intraoperatively, align a degree gauge with the marked semi-meridians. Set the knife extension to the desired depth (usually 600 µm or 90% of corneal thickness). In eyes with corneal thinning, intraoperative pachymetry can be used to avoid an incision depth of greater than 95%. We make these incisions perpendicular to the corneal surface and place them at the 9-mm zone, which is typically just central to the anterior insertion of the conjunctival vessels (Figure 4-14).

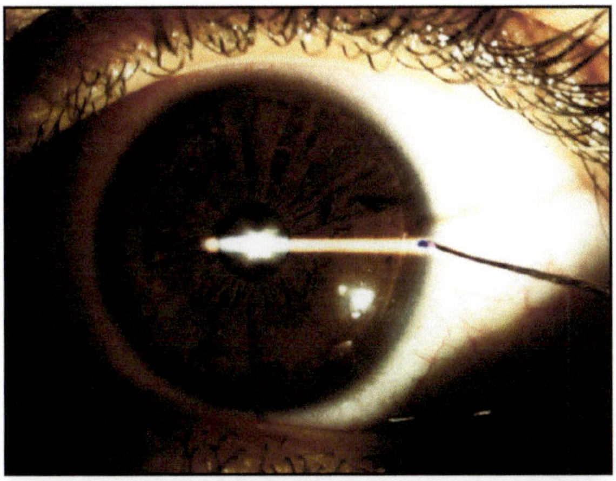

Figure 4-11. Slit-lamp marking. A thin slit beam transects the center of the pupil and crosses the limbus while a Sinskey hook stained with gentian violet dye is used to mark the corneal and conjunctival epithelia at the 180-degree semi-meridian. A mark at the 270-degree semi-meridian can also be seen.

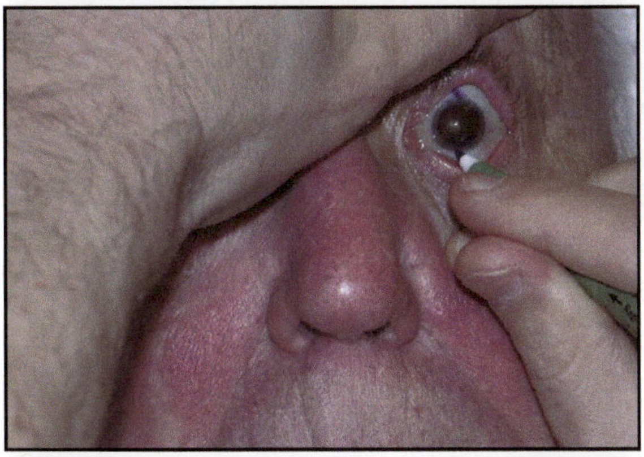

Figure 4-12. Bedside marking. While the patient is sitting in an upright position and fixating on an object directly in front of the left eye, the physician marks the corneal and conjunctival epithelia with a fine tip marking pen at the 270-degree semi-meridian. A mark at the 90-degree semi-meridian can also be seen. (Reprinted with permission of Stephen C. Pflugfelder, MD.)

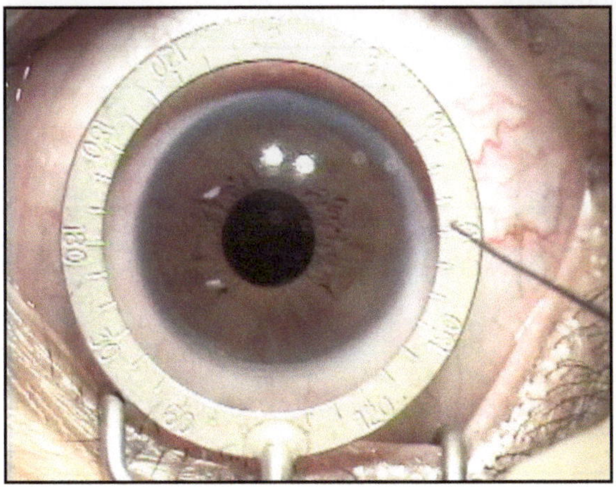

Figure 4-13. Intraoperative marking. The degree gauge is aligned with the 90- and 270-degree semi-meridians, and the steep meridian is marked with a Sinskey hook at the steep axis. Here the steep meridian is at 0 degrees.

Indications for Astigmatic Correction

In our practice, the management of astigmatism in patients undergoing cataract surgery is as follows: (1) eyes with 1.25 to 1.50 D of with-the-rule (WTR) astigmatism receive PCRIs, (2) eyes with greater than 0.40 D of against-the-rule (ATR) astigmatism receive toric intraocular lenses ([IOLs]; recent studies have shown that the posterior cornea has average of 0.30 D of ATR astigmatism),[2] (3) eyes receiving multifocal or accommodating IOLs receive PCRIs if the astigmatism is as

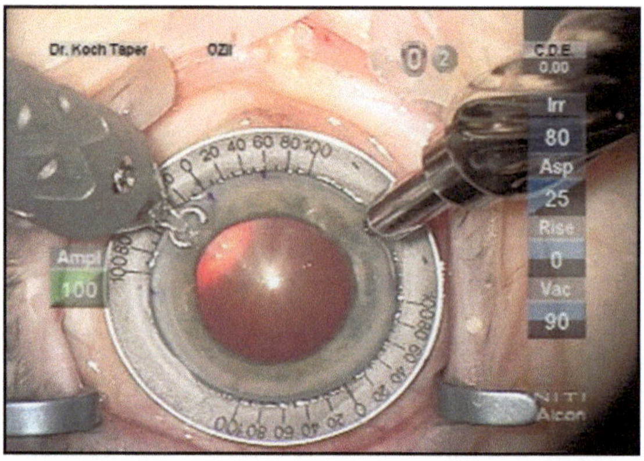

Figure 4-14. Peripheral corneal relaxing incision. The 0-degree mark on PCRI degree gauge is centered at the steep meridian. An incision is carried from one 60-degree mark to the 60-degree mark on the other side of the 0-degree mark to create an incision 60 degrees in length.

Table 4-2. Koch/Wang PCRI Nomogram for Use in Conjunction With Cataract Surgery

CATARACT: WTR ASTIGMATISM NOMOGRAM[a]

Preoperative Astigmatism (D)	*Patient Age (y)*	*Number of Incisions*	*Length (Degrees)*
1.25 to 1.75	<65	2	35 (or 1 x 50 if asymmetric)
	≥65	1	35
> 1.75 D[b]	<65	2	60
	≥65	2	45

CATARACT: ATR/OBLIQUE ASTIGMATISM NOMOGRAM[c]

Preoperative Astigmatism (D)	*Patient Age (y)*	*Number of Incisions*	*Length (Degrees)*
0.40 to 0.80	All ages	1	35 to 40
		2	30
1.26 to 1.75	All ages	1	45
		2	40
≥1.75	All ages	2	45

Combined with 2.4-mm temporal corneal incision and based on 600-μm depth.

[a]Based on corneal astigmatism.

[b]Rarely treat more than 2.00 D with PCRIs.

[c]Based on corneal astigmatism. If the cataract incision is not directly centered on the steep meridian, use a greater PCRI incision length (eg, two 30-degree PCRIs instead of one 40-degree PCRI to correct 1.25 D of astigmatism).

noted in indications 1 and 2, and (4) eyes with astigmatism too great to be fully corrected with toric IOLs may receive PCRIs at the time of surgery or, more commonly, a few weeks postoperatively to allow compensation for any unanticipated outcome of the toric IOL (Table 4-2).

We find oblique astigmatism to be a bit of a conundrum, as we suspect that many of the corneas are in the natural transition from WTR to ATR astigmatism. As a result, we treat them conservatively, use the ATR astigmatism nomograms, and, if measurements suggest 2 different steep meridians (but still not differing by more than 10 degrees), we center the incision(s) on the more horizontal of these meridians.

It is important to consider the refractive astigmatism, even when performing PCRIs in combination with cataract surgery, as the spectacle correction can provide a clue to posterior corneal astigmatism. One should be especially aware of ATR astigmatism correction in the spectacles, as this is a good indicator of total corneal astigmatism that must be addressed. Our work has shown that the posterior cornea is steep vertically and produces ATR refractive astigmatism: 0.50 D or more in corneas with anterior WTR astigmatism and 0.30 D or more in eyes with anterior ATR astigmatism.[2] Please note that this astigmatism is not accounted for by keratometers that measure only the anterior corneal curvature. Because net corneal ATR astigmatism increases over time, we target 0.25 to 0.50 D of WTR astigmatism postoperatively. We have observed that patients will tolerate an axis flip of this low magnitude.

Timing During Cataract Surgery

When combining PCRIs with cataract surgery, we prefer to place PCRIs at the conclusion of the surgery. By performing the incision at the conclusion of the surgery, the PCRI can be omitted if there was a need to enlarge the keratome incision or if the site of the keratome incision was changed. Another presumed advantage to performing the incision at the conclusion of the surgery is the theoretical lower risk of corneal perforation and avoidance of intraoperative corneal clouding at the incision site. A disadvantage of performing the PCRI at the conclusion of the surgery is the possible greater variability in intraocular pressure and in corneal thickness due to intraoperative corneal swelling, which could lead to less consistent results.

One important issue is the placement of PCRIs relative to other incisions. We prefer that they not intersect with paracentesis or keratome wounds. If needed, we place PCRIs more central or peripheral to the paracentesis wounds to avoid perforating the paracentesis roof. Posterior corneal relaxing incisions can adjoin clear corneal keratome incisions. If the nomogram calls for one incision in the meridian of the keratome incision, our preference is to make the cataract wound temporally and place the PCRI nasally.

Posterior Corneal Relaxing Incisions in Virgin and Postphotorefractive Keratectomy/Laser in Situ Keratomileusis Eyes

PCRIs are often helpful in virgin eyes or in eyes that have undergone excimer laser ablation and that have 0.50 to 2.00 D of astigmatism, with a spherical equivalent refractive error near plano (Table 4-3). PCRIs allow the surgeon to avoid the complications associated with surface ablation enhancements, such as corneal haze, and complications associated with laser in situ keratomileusis (LASIK) enhancements, such as epithelial ingrowth and a hyperopic shift, which can occur when correcting astigmatism along the flat meridian.[3-5] In eyes with prior LASIK, we avoid incising the LASIK flap.

PCRIs can be considered at 3 months after LASIK and photorefractive keratectomy (PRK) when the manifest refraction has been proven to be stable at 2 visits. In our retrospective case series studying PCRIs in 33 eyes with residual astigmatism ranging from 0.75 to 3.62 D after refractive corneal surgery, we found that the percentage of eyes within ±0.50 D increased from 0% preoperatively to 73% postoperatively, and eyes within ±1.00 D increased from 45% preoperatively to 97% postoperatively.[6]

Table 4-3. Koch/Wang Peripheral Corneal Relaxing Incision Nomogram for Patients With Naturally Occurring Astigmatism or Astigmatism After PRK or LASIK

NATURALLY OCCURRING OR AFTER PRK/LASIK: WTR ASTIGMATISM NOMOGRAM[a]

Preoperative Astigmatism (D)	*Patient Age (y)*	*Number of Incisions*	*Length (Degrees)*
0.75 to 1.00	<65	2	40
	≥65	1	45
1.01 to 1.75	<65	2	50
	≥65	2	45
>1.75	<65	2	60
	≥65	2	50

NATURALLY OCCURRING OR AFTER PRK/LASIK: ATR/OBLIQUE ASTIGMATISM NOMOGRAM[a]

Preoperative Astigmatism (D)	*Patient Age (y)*	*Number of Incisions*	*Length (Degrees)*
0.75 to 1.00	All ages	2	35 (or 1 at 40)
1.01 to 1.75	All ages	2	40
>2.00	Prefer laser enhancement		

Based on 600-µm depth and 9-mm optical zone.
[a]Based on refractive astigmatism.

Final Recommendations

1. Avoid transecting blood vessels with PCRIs, as vascular tissue promotes incisional scarring and wound contraction, causing regression of effect.
2. Avoid incisions greater than 4.5 mm in length along the horizontal or oblique meridians, as they may gape and lead to chronic foreign body sensation.
3. Be cautious in performing PCRIs in patients with dry eyes, especially along the horizontal meridian, as they can reduce corneal sensation and exacerbate dry eye symptoms.
4. Target for mild undercorrection because one can readily address undercorrections by enlarging the initial incision.

Key Points

- Quantify the astigmatism with 2 devices. One device should be a corneal topographer or Scheimpflug analyzer. The agreement between the devices should be within 0.50 D and 10 degrees.
- Compare the power and the axis from your devices to the manifest refraction and spectacle correction. If the PCRI procedure will not be combined with another surgery (eg, cataract

surgery), the refractive astigmatism quantified in the manifest refraction will trump the topographic astigmatism.

- If the PCRI will be combined with cataract surgery, spectacle correction can provide a clue to posterior corneal astigmatism. In 90% of the time, posterior corneal astigmatism contributes to ATR astigmatism and, on average, contributes 0.4 D of astigmatism.[7] As a result, the Baylor nomogram adjustment should be considered.

References

1. Swami AU, Steinert RF, Osborne WE, White AA. Rotational malposition during laser in situ keratomileusis. *Am J Ophthalmol.* 2002;133(4):561-562.
2. Koch D. *Corneal optics for IOL selection: cracking the code.* The Charles D. Kelman Innovator's Lecture. ASCRS/ASOA Symposium and Congress 2012; April 20-23, 2012; Chicago, IL.
3. Gartry DS, Larkin DF, Hill AR, Ficker LA, Steele AD. Retreatment for significant regression after excimer laser photorefractive keratectomy. A prospective, randomized, masked trial. *Ophthalmology.* 1998;105(1):131-141.
4. Perez-Santonja JJ, Ayala MJ, Sakla HF, Ruiz-Moreno JM, Alio JL. Retreatment after laser in situ keratomileusis. *Ophthalmology.* 1999;106(1):21-28.
5. Excimer laser photorefractive keratectomy (PRK) for myopia and astigmatism. American Academy of Ophthalmology. *Ophthalmology.* 1999;106(2):422-437.
6. Wang L, Swami A, Koch DD. Peripheral corneal relaxing incisions after excimer laser refractive surgery. *J Cataract Refract Surg.* 2004;30(5):1038-1044.
7. Koch DD, Ali SF, Weikert MP, Shirayama M, Jenkins R, Wang L. Contribution of posterior corneal astigmatism to total corneal astigmatism. *J Cataract Refract Surg.* 2012 Dec;38(12):2080-7.

Section 4: My Approach to Limbal Relaxing Incisions

Randall J. Olson, MD

Limbal relaxing incisions (LRIs) have been performed for a long period of time, and many surgeons have implemented this technique into their practice, whereas others have had such mixed results that they have either tried it for a short period of time, considered it, or have simply decided that this element of astigmatism correction is not important. Increasingly, however, patients are becoming more demanding of better uncorrected vision; therefore, if the surgeon ignores astigmatism, the potential of having dissatisfied patients is increased. Furthermore, with the rising cuts in third-party reimbursement for surgery, LRIs represent a potential improvement in refractive outcome that is affordable for the patient, can produce a revenue stream for the practice, and thus holds substantive value for both parties.

Many surgeons believe that use of toric intraocular lenses (IOLs) is a better answer; however, this is not an "either or" question. Toric IOLs still often result in residual refractive error, and to tweak their results, or increase their range, LRIs represent a powerful addition to help achieve a better outcome.

My approach to astigmatism surgery is to be honest about the expected results—that the goal is to decrease residual astigmatism to 0.50 diopters (D) or less; however, because I do not want to make it worse, the approach will intentionally be conservative, as one can always do more surgery. Conversely, it is difficult to reverse the astigmatism effect. By being realistic and using my actual past results, I can tell a patient with 1.00 to 1.50 D of classic astigmatism that I have an 85% chance of meeting the 0.50 D or less goal. At 2.00 D of astigmatism, this goal of getting below 0.50 D of astigmatism to 65%, and at 2.50 to 3.00 D (the realistic limit as to how much astigmatism I can attack with this technique), the odds drop to 50% when performing LRIs. However, taking a patient from 3.00 to 1.25 D of residual astigmatism is realistic, commonly achievable, and well worth the effort in uncorrected and corrected visual quality. In patients with a clear lens (potential refractive lenticular surgery and existing pseudophakic patients) or those with milder cataracts, providing trial spectacles can be helpful in demonstrating the potential visual result. If the patient has no interest, then the conversation is very brief and I move on.

My approach to the actual procedure will be outlined in the sections that follow.

Preoperative Strategy

The first question to ask is which patients are likely to be helped by LRIs? This is a decision that should be made when the patient is being evaluated for cataract or refractive lenticular surgery. Although there is much more information that may be relevant, I obtain corneal topography for those patients likely to have cataract surgery prior to placing any drops in the eye and when he or she is being evaluated for surgery, so we have a chance to discuss the options that make sense. Topography that suggests residual astigmatism would be greater than 1.00 D (up to approximately 2.50 D) points toward the role for LRIs to eliminate or vastly decrease the patient's total amount of astigmatism. It has also been my experience that with-the-rule or against-the-rule astigmatism does better, whereas oblique astigmatism seems to be less effectively treated with LRIs.[1] I believe this may be due to lid position because on slit-lamp examination after surgery, I can see the lid position often closing these incisions on postoperative day 1. I would like for other surgeons to report their results on oblique astigmatism to determine whether they have similar findings.

All of these issues are taken into consideration when discussing whether astigmatism should be considered for correction. This discussion need not be lengthy. I cover (1) the need, (2) the expected result (always under-promise so that delivery is usually exceeded), and (3) the expected complications. I have never had a major complication; however, I do mention wound melt and infection to the patient. It is important to point out that irritation, especially for those with dry eye syndrome, is common and that the dry eye condition can be exacerbated. In fact, severe dry eye is a contraindication for this procedure. The patient is then taken to a refractive coordinator to discuss further the option he or she might want to undergo, as well as to discuss the cost. This is also my approach with toric IOLs as well.

When the decision has been made to perform LRIs, it is important to acquire all of the relevant information, which would include a follow-up topography where there have been no drops placed in the eye (often on the day of surgery), as well as the biometry and the patient's refractive error. Of the three, the refractive error is the least important in that cataracts can induce lenticular astigmatism; however, I am most confident when all 3 agree relatively closely in regard to the amount and axis of astigmatism. Remember, refractive cylinder is typically only 70% of what one will note on topography, so that difference is to be expected. I am particularly concerned when there is obvious irregular astigmatism or lack of agreement between either of the 2 topographies, or the topography and biometry. This is a red flag that there might be other issues and would be a reason to wait until after the primary surgery to perform LRIs, which easily can be carried out in a minor-procedure room. Most of the time, however, in appropriately screened patients, it is clear that astigmatism correction can be offered, planned, and surgically repaired.

One large group of which to be concerned are those who have significant lid disease or dry eye syndrome. LRIs can definitely exacerbate, and at times substantially exacerbate, these patients' symptoms; therefore, I am reluctant to offer this procedure in those individuals who have dry eye syndrome, meibomian gland dysfunction, or blepharitis that is not well-controlled. In fact, in these instances, if the patient really wants astigmatism correction, I tend to lean toward toric lens implantation and not incisional correction.

My approach to surgical planning and nomogram use is simple, is based on my historic information, and is similar to what Dr. Kevin Miller has presented for a long time (Table 4-4). Our published results[1] show that this nomogram is conservative, resulting in few overcorrections, and it

Table 4-4. My Astigmatism Nomogram Based on Dr. Kevin Miller's Approach
• Make the cataract incision on the minor or major cylinder axis so that axis rotation is minimized.
• If the cataract incision is on the steep axis (usually against-the-rule astigmatism), then subtract 0.25 D from the total amount of cylinder. Conversely, add 0.25 D if the incision is on the flat axis (usually with-the-rule astigmatism). This is the amount to be corrected.
• The LRI is centered on the steep axis and is 60 degrees in length for every diopter of astigmatism. For any astigmatism more than 1.00 D, it is best to split the amount equally on both sides of the steep axis.
• Do not do more than 90 degrees of LRI in any meridian! This means that up to 3.00 D theoretically can be corrected, but our average results are less than this.
• Avoid temporal LRIs that cross the main incision. I prefer adding these after surgery when the incision is stable and astigmatism results are clearly known.

is easy to calculate. Essentially, with-the-rule or against-the-rule astigmatism is treated differently in that I always approach these patients temporally and will vary my incisions slightly to try to be "on-axis" in either the minor or major astigmatic meridian so not to induce much axis shift with my cataract incision. My overall format is that I look at the astigmatism axis, and if it is with-the-rule, I need to correct approximately 0.25 D more than is recorded through topography; against-the-rule is corrected approximately 0.25 D less (owing to the surgically induced component from my main penetrating temporal phaco incision). For the majority of patients between the ages of 55 and 85, I have not noted a statistically significant difference based on age,[1] so I treat all such patients the same, which is essentially 0.50 D of correction per 30 degrees of incision. I map out this information, record it in the biometry chart, and determine the surgical plan while in the preoperative area. For example, if I know that I need to make a 2.00-D correction at the 90-degree axis (meaning that the topography was approximately 1.75 D at the 90-degree axis), correction would require 120 degrees of incision, which I would split equally into 2 60-degree incisions. I think the important point here is to make the procedure as simple as possible because the more complicated we make it, the more it keeps surgeons from embracing it.

Performing the Limbal Relaxing Incision

I have worked with Mr. Doug Mastel to compose a set of instruments that have worked well in my hands (Figure 4-15). These instruments are available from Mastel Precision Ophthalmic Surgical Instruments Inc, and I have no financial interest in them. Essentially, the instruments include a guide ring with an angled internal edge that when placed on the cornea will result in a peripheral arcuate clear corneal incision at an optical zone of 10 mm, and if the blade is run exactly along the internal aspect of the guide, the incision will be made perpendicular to the corneal surface and will always be exactly semicircular. The blade is diamond and makes a 600-µm cut if run evenly along the epithelium. Precision, especially perpendicularity, are important aspects for consistent results. I feel that increased intraocular pressure (IOP) causes these incisions to gape, which is the same as adding tissue to the steep meridian, until they fill in with epithelium and then scar tissue. This gape will be greatest for an incision that is exactly perpendicular to the corneal surface, and if the incision is beveled (ie, not perpendicular), the IOP will close the incision so there will be

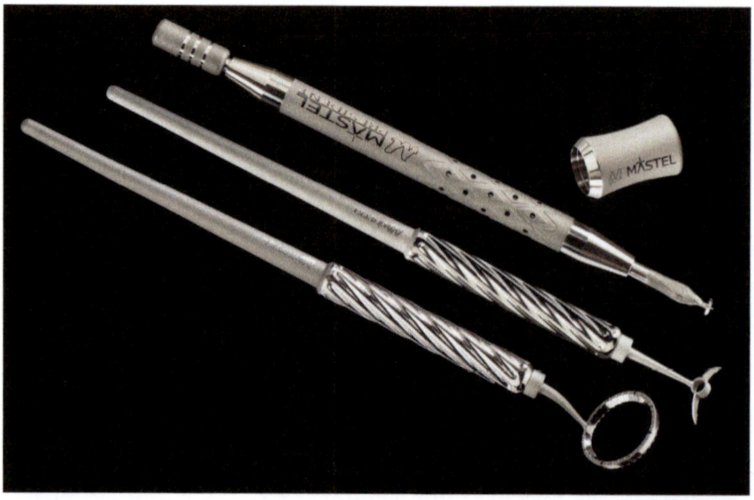

Figure 4-15. A customized set of instruments for performing limbal relaxing incisions made by Mastel Precision Ophthalmic Surgical Instruments Inc. The guide is made to create a 10.0-mm optical zone and the blade, if run precisely against the edge of the guide, will guarantee a semi-circular incision that is 600 μm deep and perpendicular to the corneal surface. (Reprinted with permission from Mastel Precision.)

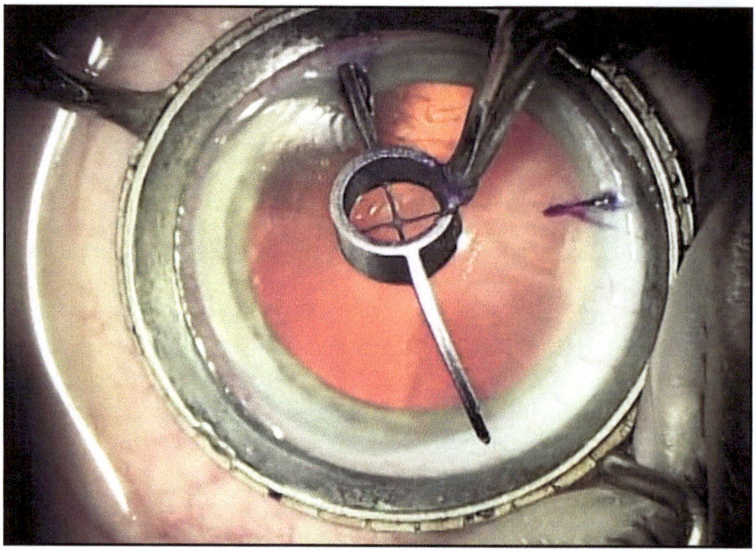

Figure 4-16. With the guide lined up on the 0- to 180-degree meridian, the steep axis is noted and the degrees of incision are marked with dye and a marker. To avoid any confusion, it is best to clearly write this information on a topography printout and have it visible at the start of the procedure.

less effect. I have seen many so-called LRI failures where it is apparent that the incisions were not close to perpendicular, and I feel this is a common cause of failure.

Therefore, my approach to LRIs is as follows:

1. Mark the steep axis. My experience in marking these patients is that in individuals aged 50 years and older, cyclotorsion while in the recumbent position is minimal to nonexistent; therefore, I have stopped marking patients in the upright position prior to lying down if they are 50 years or older. However, it is important to mark younger patients in the upright position. In cataract surgery patients, LRIs are the first step of the surgery. I start by lining up the ring, which is marked in 10-degree increments, on the 0 to 180 degree meridian. Noting any feature of the iris or limbus, such as an iris nevus or limbal vascular structure, from a previous slit-lamp examination helps with this step. The topography chart with notes indicated should be nearby so there is no question about the steep axis and the amount of surgery, which is carefully noted; then, the degrees of incision are marked on the cornea with dye on a marker (Figure 4-16). Write this information out clearly on a topography map ahead of time so there is no confusion. If 60 degrees of incision at axis 90 is the goal, then locate the 90-degree meridian and count off 30 degrees (3 marks on the instrument I use) on each side and mark them.

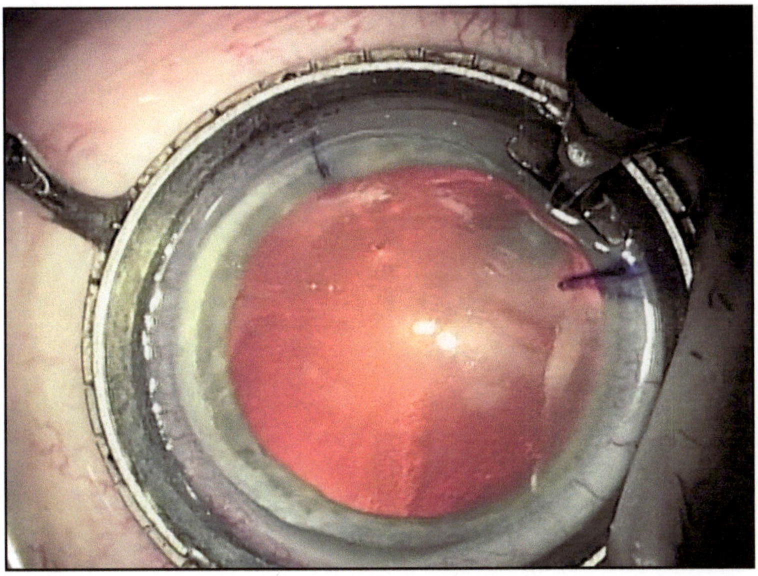

Figure 4-17. The blade is started in one of the marks against the guide and continued to the second mark, making sure that the blade is snug against the guide throughout. The diamond blade carrier is run along the epithelial surface to make the 600-µm deep cut. Also, make sure the blade is not torqued to either side or a less deep cut will result. Do not push the blade into the stroma or corneal perforation is possible.

I have seen many errors (working on the flat meridian for instance—not a good idea!) related to not having this clearly outlined in writing and hanging on a wall or on a clipboard for easy reference, especially for a beginner surgeon.

2. Making the incisions. The knife itself is a diamond blade that cuts 600 µm if lightly held against the epithelial surface. The blade is inserted at one of the outside marks for the incision, right up against the edge of the guide, and I make sure that I am snug against its internal edge. With the blade well seated into the cornea, it is then advanced along the guide to the opposite mark, always guaranteeing a 600-µm deep incision that is circular (Figure 4-17). Take special care to be along the guide edge so that you are perpendicular to the surface, and do not have the blade torqued to either side against the guide, as this would decrease the depth of the cut and could impact the results. This process is then carried out on the opposite side. I use my left hand to hold the LRI knife when working on the left side of the eye, and my right hand on the opposite side. I tend to use my right hand for more nasal (using a temporal surgical approach) incision and my left hand for more temporal incisions; however, this should depend on what is most comfortable for the surgeon. I then take my irrigating solution bottle with a blunt cannula tip, open the incisions, irrigate, and feel along the entire incision to make sure that I am equally deep throughout (Figure 4-18). This actually may help gape and stretch the incision slightly, and it helps to make sure that my result is exactly as I want it. It is easy to touch up an area where you think you are not quite as deep as you should be; however, with experience, this is rarely necessary. I have never perforated an eye; however, to avoid perforation, it is critical not to push on the corneal surface, especially if touching up an area, because the instrument can easily slide into the incision and make a deeper and potentially penetrating cut if not careful.

Other Special Considerations

For patients with against-the-rule astigmatism, I have had a few leaky wounds, which are at high risk for endophthalmitis[2] for which I have made a temporal LRI and then my own cataract incision through this. Therefore, I tend to avoid temporal relaxing incisions if I cannot avoid my main incision, and alternatively go up to 90 degrees with a single nasal incision that will correct

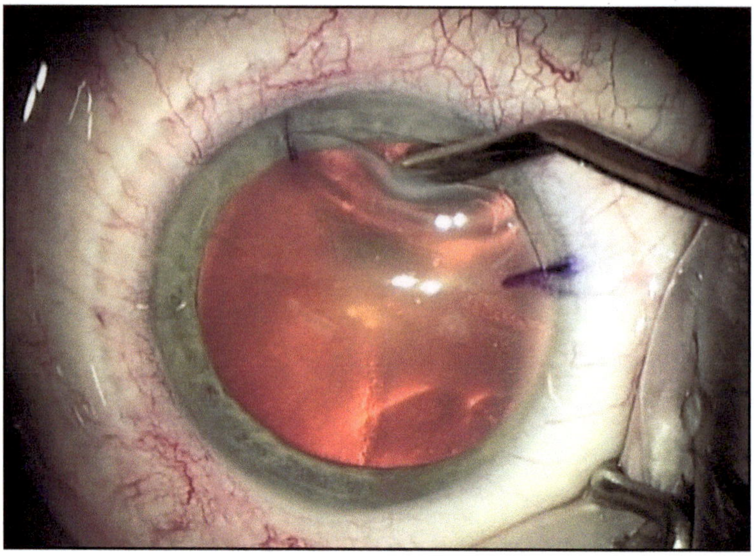

Figure 4-18. The blunt irrigation cannula is placed into the resulting incision(s), the incision is irrigated, and the depth of the incision is checked throughout the entire length. If an area is shallow, this can be easily touched up with the diamond blade; however, be very light with a second pass because corneal perforation is now a greater risk because the incision is already made and can easily gape.

up to 2.00 D of astigmatism when including the main cataract incision into the mix. If I need more touch up, I will add a temporal relaxing incision later, after the primary surgery. It is interesting how often there is more correction than one would expect, and I have seen up to 2.50 D corrected in this manner, so it has been an effective approach and has obviated any concern about the incisions leaking. When in doubt of incision security, I always place a suture for at least 1 week, which may reduce the LRI effect, at least temporarily, so waiting until later for a touch-up has been a good compromise for me.

Because I often will do LRI touch-ups in the minor procedure room after primary surgery, my general rule is to never do more than 2 90-degree incisions that are 180 degrees apart overall to avoid an unstable cornea which, fortunately, I have never seen. However, one exception is a touch up 1 year or more later, where the original incisions look well healed. I believe we get a second chance to further correct up to 1.50 D, even if 180 degrees of total incision has already been performed, particularly in patients where overcorrection is an issue, in that these additional incisions will be placed in untouched territory. If conservatively approached as described herein, overcorrection is a rare problem other than small in degrees.[1] Postoperatively, I treat these cases with topical antibiotics 4 times a day for 1 week, as I do with my regular cataract surgery patients, and I suggest to the patient that he or she should use frequent artificial tears as needed for symptoms. I also tell my patients that they will have some scratchiness for several weeks. Other than in those with significant dry eye or lid disease, it is a surprisingly minimal postoperative problem.

Postoperative Complications

Other than dry eye symptoms, I have not had any significant complications. I have never had a perforation after having performed thousands of these incisions; however, I have had significant increase in dry eye symptoms in those with underlying dry eye problems. This is the only substantial issue or problem that I have encountered. Because my approach is conservative, and, as mentioned, overcorrection has been uncommon (usually occurring only in patients who are more than 80 years of age), I have become more conservative in my overall approach. I have cut back my surgery to approximately two-thirds of the amount listed in the nomogram for those 85 years or older and have not seen an overcorrection since then.

Another group to be concerned about are those patients who have less than 1.00 D of cylinder. Our published study[1] showed that results are more erratic in these individuals, with overcorrection more likely to occur and topography accuracy more variable. You can often tell when such cases will be a problem, that is when topography is not consistent from one examination to the next, or when there are differences between refraction, topography, and IOL biometry/keratometry. When in doubt, it is always best to wait until after the primary surgery, as LRIs may easily be performed as an enhancement procedure following healing and documentation of a stable and accurate refractive state.

Conclusion

LRIs are a very easy and forgiving approach to astigmatism correction that is added to other approaches for astigmatism control. For those with 1.50 D or less of astigmatism, LRIs are quite accurate and can also be effective for even more cylinder (up to 3.00 D in my experience), with the understanding that residual astigmatism becomes more common the higher we go. To get patients within 0.50 D, LRIs is a very powerful approach and has resulted in many happy patients with a minimal amount of concern and complications.

Key Points

- Be conservative because you can always do more, but it is hard to undo an overcorrection.
- Write out the surgical plan on a copy of the topography and post it where it is visible at the time of surgery.
- Wait if astigmatism measurements show inconsistency for either axis or amount of cylinder.
- For patients 50 years or older, cyclotorsion is minimal and the steep axis can be marked with the patient in the recumbent position.

References

1. Bradley MJ, Coombs J, Olson RJ. Analysis of an approach to astigmatism correction during cataract surgery. *Ophthalmologica*. 2006;220(5):311-316.
2. Wallin T, Parker J, Jin Y, Kefalopoulos G, Olson RJ. Cohort study of 27 cases of endophthalmitis at a single institution. *J Cataract Refract Surg*. 2005;31(4):735-741.

Section 5: My Guide to Peripheral Corneal Relaxing Incisions

Jonathan B. Rubenstein, MD

Patients presenting for cataract surgery today are not only expecting improved vision; they are also expecting spectacle independence. These high patient expectations have increased the demand for surgeons to minimize postoperative refractive error. Correction of spherical error is achieved by choosing the correct intraocular lens (IOL) power based on the determination of accurate axial length and the correct corneal power. Corneal astigmatism is another refractive error that the cataract surgeon must manage and minimize to achieve postoperative emmetropia. For true spectacle independence, $\leq$0.50 diopters (D) of astigmatism after surgery is required.

Options for reducing corneal astigmatism at the time of cataract surgery vary, and surgeons need to adopt one of multiple approaches based on the amount of preoperative corneal astigmatism and patient-specific considerations. This chapter will describe my approach to the correction of corneal astigmatism at the time of cataract surgery using peripheral corneal relaxing incisions (PCRIs).

Preoperative Refractive Evaluation

The first step to managing astigmatism is a comprehensive preoperative assessment. This must account for the magnitude of astigmatism, location of the axis of cylinder, patient age, and the refractive status of the other eye. To aim for spectacle independence, I will treat preoperative corneal astigmatism ≥0.75 D.

Several methods are available for evaluating astigmatic refractive error. Preoperative assessment begins with the manifest refraction to determine total astigmatism, which includes both lenticular and corneal astigmatism. Because lenticular astigmatism is eliminated with the removal of the cataractous lens, only the correction of cornel astigmatism is necessary in surgery. Therefore, accurate assessment of preoperative corneal astigmatism is needed. Manual keratometry, partial coherence interferometry (IOLMaster; Carl Zeiss Meditec Inc), optical low-coherence reflectometry (LENSTAR; Haag-Streit USA), corneal topography, and corneal elevation mapping may be utilized to assess corneal astigmatism. Each surgeon must determine which preoperative test provides the most accurate information in his or her hands. It is important to measure both the corneal power or the magnitude of the astigmatism and the direction or axis of astigmatism. In my experience, the magnitude of the astigmatism is most accurately assessed using manual keratometry. I personally perform keratometry on each of my preoperative cataract patients using the Bausch & Lomb manual keratometer (catalogue #71-21-35). I realize this may sound cumbersome; however, I believe an accurate assessment of corneal power is essential for obtaining reliable preoperative values. By personally performing the keratometry, I can monitor the patient's fixation and centration. Therefore, I can evaluate the validity of the keratometry. Performing keratometry yourself also allows for the discovery of irregular astigmatism. If the mires are not round, wavy, or distorted, this indicates the presence of an irregular corneal surface, which can decrease the accuracy of the keratometry values. If the mires do not superimpose, this may indicate irregular astigmatism from an irregular corneal shape, such as that due to corneal warpage or keratoconus. Therefore, by performing keratometry yourself, you can assess the health and regularity of the cornea and also determine the validity of your measurements. To determine the proper astigmatic axis, I utilize the quantitative axis determination from the IOLMaster keratometry values. If the 3 readings are within 0.25 D in power and within 5 degrees in axis, I find that the axis location is accurate. It is also important to obtain topographic corneal maps and corneal elevation maps to use as a qualitative guide for axis determination. These corneal mapping tests also help to expose irregular astigmatism and corneal shape abnormalities. The quantitative axis that is determined by the IOLMaster must be supported by the axis found on corneal maps.

Therefore, in summary, I feel that the best assessment of corneal power is derived from careful manual keratometry, and the best assessment of astigmatic axis is derived from the IOLMaster interferometer keratometries combined with qualitative guidance from corneal topography and corneal elevation mapping.

Preoperative Planning

Before taking a patient to the operating room, it is essential to create a preoperative plan. This should be done in the office well in advance of the day of surgery. For astigmatism management, the precise surgical technique should be planned out and written in the chart. When using PCRIs,

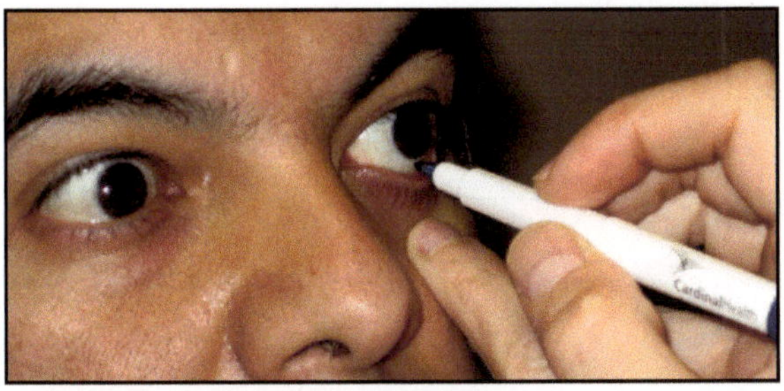

Figure 4-19. Marking the 6-o'clock limbus with both eyes open while fixating on the distance.

the exact location of these incisions, the length of the incisions, and the depth of the incisions must be planned. To determine the exact surgical plan, the surgeon needs to consult a nomogram. Multiple nomograms are available that determine the number of incisions and length of the incisions based on the measured amount of preoperative corneal astigmatism, the age of the patient, and the desired refractive effect. When first starting with PCRIs, it is best to plan the procedure using multiple nomograms. Eventually, with experience, you can determine which nomogram works best in your hands. With further experience, you can modify these nomograms based on your own results. I utilize both Dr. Louis D. "Skip" Nichamin's and Dr. Douglas D. Koch's fixed-blade depth nomograms for a 600-µm diamond knife. I then will modify these nomograms based on my technique. Both of these nomograms assume a clear corneal temporal cataract incision and PCRIs made with a 600-µm double-cutting diamond knife.

The exact location of the incisions must also be planned preoperatively and written in the patient's chart. The patient's peripheral cornea should be carefully examined at the slit lamp to make sure there is no evidence of corneal thinning or scarring at the planned site of the incisions. Peripheral corneal pathology could increase the chance of corneal perforations when performing the peripheral incisions.

Intraoperative Management

It is important to take the patient's chart to the operating room on the day of surgery. In the chart, the exact plan for peripheral corneal incisions should be clearly mapped out. This should include the number of incisions, the length of the incisions, and the exact axis on which these incisions are placed. For example, I will notate "Plan PCRIs: (45 degrees x 2) at 105 degrees" and write this in the patient's chart, just under the planned IOL power. The patient's cornea then needs to be marked to provide accurate alignment of the incisions. In the preoperative area, a single reference mark is placed at the 6 o'clock-position on the limbus with a fine tipped marker with the patient keeping both eyes open and fixating on my nose (Figure 4-19). It is important to have the patient sitting upright with both eyes open to avoid cyclotorsion. Although I have tried many techniques for preoperative marking of the cornea, including marking the 3- and 9-o'clock positions, I find a single mark at the 6-o'clock position is the easiest on the patient and provides the highest degree of accuracy. Then, after the patient is prepped and draped and in a supine position in the operating room, this 6-o'clock mark is used as a reference point to help mark the steep axis of astigmatism. Multiple marking systems can be employed. Again, I've tried multiple systems to mark the steep axis, but I find that the Dell astigmatic marker (Rhein Medical Ophthalmic Surgical Instruments) works best in my hands. The Dell marker is a combination of an astigmatic dial peripherally with an internal bezel with raised ridges that create 40-, 60-, and 80-degree marks on the cornea (Figure 4-20). This marker is inked with a fine-tipped surgical marker and is then applied with moderate pressure to the patient's cornea by aligning the 90-degree point on the astigmatic dial with the 6-o'clock limbal mark. Care must be taken to align the marker with the corneal limbus

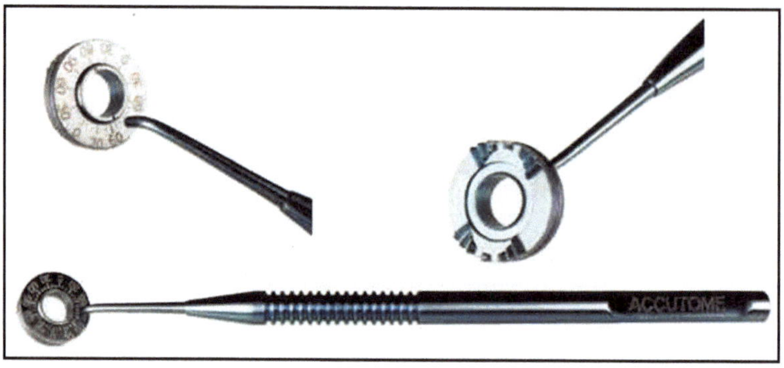

Figure 4-20. Dell-style astigmatic marker with external astigmatic dial and internal bezel. (Reprinted with permission from Accutome.)

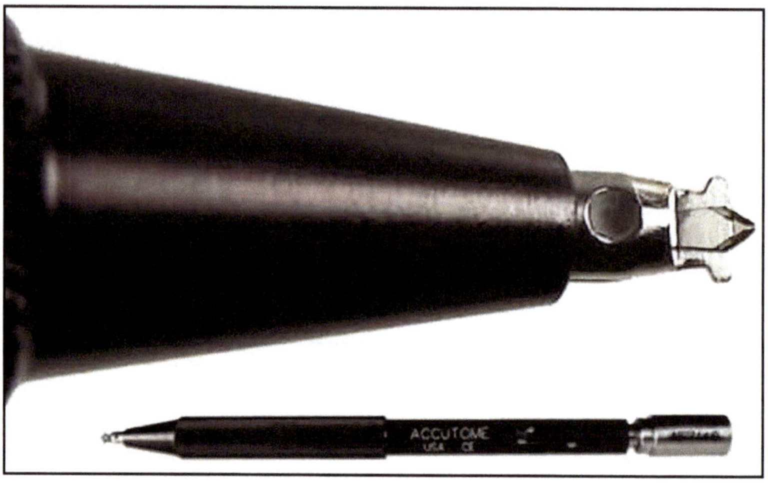

Figure 4-21. Preset, 600-µm, black diamond knife. (Reprinted with permission from Accutome.)

so it is well-centered over the cornea. The axis of steep astigmatism is dialed into the marker by rotating the internal bezel until an arrow on the bezel is aligned with the steep axis–degree mark on the outer astigmatic dial.

Surgical Technique

It is best to make the corneal incisions at the beginning of the surgical procedure because the cornea and the corneal epithelium are still clear and smooth. Also, the intraocular pressure is still controlled and within normal range. After the eyelid speculum is inserted, the cornea is marked with the inked astigmatic marker to clearly delineate the location of the steep axis and to provide degree marks that will guide the length of the incisions. A number of excellent diamond knives are available for PCRIs. These knives are generally divided into 2 categories: preset depth knives and adjustable depth knives. The blade length of the adjustable depth knives are set based on measured intraoperative peripheral corneal pachymetry. The preset diamond knives are available in depths of 550 and 600 µm. Because the peripheral cornea, in a normal state, is uniformly thicker than 600 µm, a preset knife blade should not perforate a normal peripheral cornea. It is important to choose a nomogram that is based on either the use of a preset or a pachymetry-adjusted diamond blade. Although a pachymetry-adjusted blade and nomogram potentially offers more precise results, I operate in a university hospital setting that handles 30 operating rooms' worth of equipment each day. Therefore, I cannot trust that my diamond knives are going to be cared for properly. For that reason, I use a preset, 600-µm, black diamond blade because it is less expensive to replace if damaged. I currently use a preset, 600-µm, diamond blade made by Accutome Inc (Figure 4-21).

The incisions can be made by either pushing or pulling the double-cutting diamond blade. I will rehearse the motion of cutting the incisions before actually creating the incisions, and I choose the direction of my blade movement based on the anatomy of the patient's face, nose, and forehead. Therefore, I will either push or pull the blade depending on which movement is most comfortable. For against-the-rule astigmatism incisions, because I sit temporally, I will make both incisions with my dominant hand. For with-the-rule astigmatism incisions, I will make one incision with my dominant hand and the second incision with my nondominant hand. I use a 0.12 forceps for fixating the globe by either placing one of teeth within the paracentesis incision or by grabbing the episclera near the limbus. It is important to create these incisions at the proper depth. Poor technique in creating these incisions is probably the major reason why some surgeons experience consistent undercorrections and variability with their results. The blade must remain perpendicular to the corneal surface, with adequate pressure to allow the blade to reach 90% of the measured corneal depth. Therefore, a 600-μm blade should ideally cut 540 μm into the cornea. The knife should be held with 3 fingers in the same hand position that one would use to throw a dart. When creating the incisions, care should be taken to make sure that the blade is gently rotated in the surgeon's fingertips to maintain a perpendicular angle of attack. Perpendicularity to the cornea should be maintained in the X and Y axes.

Two important caveats should be mentioned:

1. If the patient has against-the-rule astigmatism, and the planned peripheral corneal incision is coincident with the clear corneal (temporal) cataract incision, the PCRI should be limited to a 3-mm length. The clear corneal cataract incision is then made within this PCRI in a 2-plane fashion by entering the cornea at a 50% depth within the relaxing incision. If the nomogram calls for a PCRI that is longer than 3 mm, the against-the-rule astigmatism incisions can be lengthened at the end of surgery once the lens implant is in place and the eye is still filled with viscoelastic to maintain a normal pressure. Keeping the original temporal relaxing incision at 3 mm or less prevents the cataract incision from extending and tearing during the manipulation of phacoemulsification. If the peripheral corneal incision does extend from excessive phaco handpiece manipulation, this incision may leak and require suturing.

2. If the nomogram requires a with-the-rule astigmatism incision, it is important to make sure that the paracentesis incision does not interfere with the peripheral corneal incision. It is best to make the PCRI slightly more central and the paracentesis incision more peripheral. This avoids tearing and stretching of the peripheral corneal incision that may occur if the PCRIs intersect the paracentesis incisions.

Aside from these 2 considerations, phacoemulsification cataract surgery should proceed normally. The power of the lens implant does not have to be altered when PCRIs are used. For every 1 D of corneal flattening at the axis of the incision, there is 1 D of corneal steepening 90 degrees away, leaving overall spherical neutrality.

Complications

Fortunately, complications associated with PCRIs are rare. The most common complication would be either undercorrection or overcorrection. This can be remedied either by extending the relaxing incisions or by excimer laser surgery after the postoperative refraction becomes stable. Corneal perforation can occur, but it is quite uncommon. The usual causes for corneal perforation include unrecognized peripheral corneal thinning—a diamond blade abnormality secondary to excessive protrusion of the blade—or tearing of the incisions from manipulation in surgery. If a perforation is recognized, the leaky incisions must be sutured until the incisions are watertight. The sutures can be removed in the postoperative period by titrating their removal based on measured postoperative astigmatism. Infection is also quite rare. Care should be taken to treat blepharitis in the preoperative period to minimize the chance of bacterial exposure to the corneal incisions.

Conclusion

Peripheral corneal relaxing incisions are a useful and effective method of minimizing postoperative corneal astigmatism. This technique can be quite predictable if performed in a careful and compulsive fashion. Even with the availability of excellent toric IOL implants, PCRIs will always have a place in our surgical armamentarium. These incisions provide a less expensive alternative to toric lenses and can also be used as an adjunct to toric lens implants in patients with high astigmatic corrections. Finally, when patients do not have intact capsular bags, PCRIs can effectively reduce astigmatism when a 3-piece IOL implant is placed in the ciliary sulcus or secured with anterior capsule capture.

Key Points

- The best preoperative method for the assessment of the *magnitude* of corneal astigmatism is manual keratometry.
- The best preoperative method for the quantitative assessment of the *axis* of corneal astigmatism is the IOLMaster, with qualitative guidance from corneal topography.
- I suggest that the cataract surgeon perform his or her own manual keratometry.
- The surgical plan for PCRIs should be created preoperatively, written in the patient's chart, and brought to the operating room.
- Good surgical technique is critical for good results. The surgical blade needs to be set with adequate pressure to achieve optimal depth, and the blade must remain perpendicular to the cornea for the entire incision.
- Limit the PCRI incision to a 3-mm length when the axis is *against-the-rule* and is coincident with the clear corneal temporal cataract wound. Extend the incision only after the phacoemulsification is done and the lens implant is in position.
- Avoid the intersection of the paracentesis incision with the PCRIs when the axis is *with-the-rule.*

Section 6: Astigmatism in Three Dimensions

R. Bruce Wallace III, MD

Reducing corneal astigmatism is essential for successful refractive lens replacement procedures, commonly known as refractive cataract surgery (RCS), and limbal relaxing incisions (LRIs) are one of the friendliest and most cost effective refractive procedures we can offer our patients. With a LRI procedure, there is no expensive laser, no central corneal or intraocular trauma, and perforations are rare in healthy corneas. So why are not many cataract surgeons yet using LRIs? Some surgeons are not convinced they are reliable. For many, the awkwardness of incisional corneal surgery, along with an uncomfortable change in routine for surgeon and staff, has placed LRIs in a negative light. Yet, judging by the swell in attendance at teaching events like Dr. Louis D. "Skip" Nichamin's LRI wet labs at the past few American Academy of Ophthalmology and American Society of Cataract and Refractive Surgery meetings, LRI popularity is growing.

We owe a great deal of thanks to early pioneers who promoted the benefits of combining astigmatic keratotomy with cataract surgery decades ago. I have had the pleasure to teach LRI techniques for more than 20 years. During these training sessions, I have learned important steps to help convince cataract surgeons that LRIs can be an important part of RCS. Before a surgeon transitions to the routine use of LRIs, he or she must understand the benefits, be confident in the "system" of treatment, and be confident with his or her technique.

Astigmatism in Three Dimensions

To reduce unwanted astigmatism, the surgeon must lead the way in his or her practice to develop a systematic approach to astigmatic correction. Reducing astigmatism begins with reliable preoperative evaluation. Most cataract surgeons depend on trained technicians to perform preoperative astigmatism measurements, which include refraction, keratometry, and corneal topography. Unfortunately, many technicians do not think about astigmatism in 3 dimensions because these measurements generate only numbers or 2-dimensional color maps. For technicians and surgeons to be effective in astigmatism control, it is helpful to understand and visualize astigmatism, especially corneal astigmatism, in 3 dimensions. Terms such as the *flat meridian*, the *steep meridian axis*, the *cylinder axis*, and *coupling* become easier to grasp when thinking of corneal shapes, rather than numbers or colors.

To determine whether your office staff perceives astigmatism in 3 dimensions, try this experiment. Ask your best trained technicians to imagine that the oblong curvatures of an American football represent the astigmatic corneal surfaces of a patient's eye, with the curvature along one meridian being steep and the other flat. Imagine that the football is lying flat on the ground. Would it resemble with-the-rule or against-the-rule astigmatism? If the technicians answer with-the-rule astigmatism, they are correct and are probably thinking about astigmatism in 3 dimensions. With this fundamental understanding of what the term *regular astigmatism* means, all members of the surgical team will find astigmatism correction easier to understand.

Surgical Planning

The goal for astigmatism control should be the creation of a resultant cylinder of less than 1.00 diopter (D) at any axis. Most patients enjoy good unaided visual acuity with this degree of astigmatism. Some studies suggest a benefit to leaving some amount of residual against-the-rule cylinder so that uncorrected near vision after cataract surgery is improved.[1] However, surgical practices utilizing multifocal intraocular lenses (IOLs) and/or monovision will not find this to be an advantage because of the compromise of loss of distance visual acuity with amounts more than 1.00 D of cylinder.[2]

One of the more challenging tasks that a surgeon faces is deciding which astigmatic preoperative measurements should be used when planning a surgical correction. Do we depend on the cylinder diopters and axis from the refraction or the keratometry, and do we always need to perform corneal topography? One study showed the frequency of poor correlation of all 3 methods of measurement, especially with less than 2.00 D of astigmatism.[3] Fortunately, unlike correction of spherical refractive errors, astigmatism correction is more forgiving, especially when treating moderate-to-low levels.

My routine for determining placement of LRIs involves comparing IOLMaster 500 version 7.3 keratometry (Carl Zeiss Meditec Inc) with Humphrey Atlas corneal topography (Carl Zeiss Meditec Inc). If there is less than 0.75 D with-the-rule cylinder or less than 1.00 D against-the-rule cylinder, astigmatic correction is not usually added to the lens procedure. Also, if there is a poor correlation of keratometry to corneal topography or if the topography shows irregularity,

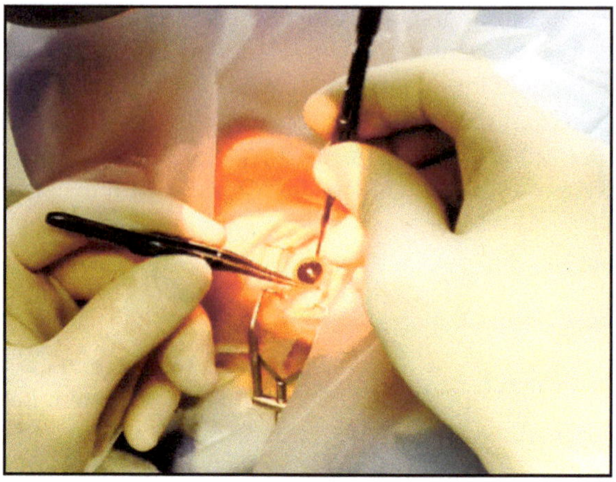

Figure 4-22. Performing opposite eye LRI.

especially inferior corneal steepening, LRIs will be delayed until postoperative topography and refraction appear regular and stable. It is not uncommon for us to perform LRIs on such eyes on the same day that we perform the RCS on the fellow eye.[4] We simply prep both eyes, and after the lens procedure on the second eye, we remove the drapes, adjust the microscope over the first eye, and reach over to perform the LRI (Figure 4-22).

A systematic approach to using LRIs improves results. A number of LRI nomograms have been developed by Gills, Lindstrom, Nichamin, and me. I first used Dr. Nichamin's nomogram and then modified it to slant more toward one incision for lower levels of cylinder (Table 4-5).

For many years, I always performed paired LRIs, which was a carryover from the 6-mm optical zone astigmatic keratotomies performed during the radial keratotomy era. I began using a single LRI after examining a 15 year old who had experienced a single partial peripheral corneal laceration that corrected his 2.00-D corneal astigmatism that was still present in his fellow eye. I found that because we make the LRI so far into the corneal periphery, single incisions do not create significant irregular astigmatism.

Because corneal diameters vary and we make arcs, not straight-line incisions, degree measurements are universally more accurate. For some surgeons, planning LRIs with computer programs has become popular, similar to the toric IOL calculator offered by Alcon Laboratories. In fact, the Abbott Medical Optics LRI calculator (http://www.LRIcalculator.com) designed by Dr. Eric Donnenfeld and the PalmScan AP2000 (MicroMedical Devices Inc) modified by Dr. Rafi Israel are now available.

Some surgeons concerned about cyclotropia will mark the 6- and 3- or 9-o'clock limbal axis at the slit lamp prior to surgery. However, this may offer little benefit for lower levels of astigmatism. Yet, for higher levels of astigmatism (more than 2.00 D), marking the limbus may be worthwhile. The Bakewell marker (Mastel Precision Ophthalmic Surgical Instruments), an instrument used to mark the horizontal axis while the patient is sitting upright in the preoperative area, may be more convenient then marking at the slit lamp.

Questions may arise concerning IOL power modifications with LRIs. With low to moderate levels of cylinder (0.50 to 2.75 D), corneal "coupling" equalizes the central cornea power, so there is less chance the IOL power selection will be inaccurate. Longer LRI incisions for higher cylinder (>3.00 D) may create a radial keratotomy effect and produce unwanted postoperative hyperopia. Increasing the IOL power 0.50 to 1.00 D may be necessary in these cases.

Similar to the preoperative discussion with patients about new refractive IOLs, informing patients about the option of surgical treatment for astigmatism has become more common in many cataract practices. I start by describing the optical disadvantages of astigmatism and the relative effectiveness and low risk surrounding LRIs. In the United States, when charging most

Table 4-5. Nomogram[a]					
WITH-THE-RULE AND OBLIQUE ASTIGMATISM					
Astigmatism (D)	*40 to 50 yo*	*50 to 60 yo*	*60 to 70 yo*	*70 to 80 yo*	*80+ yo*
1.00 to 1.50	60 degrees (1)	50 degrees (1)	50 degrees (1)	40 degrees (1)	30 degrees (1)
1.50 to 2.00	70 degrees (1)	70 degrees (1)	70 degrees (1)	60 degrees (1)	60 degrees (1)
2.00 to 2.50	60 degrees (2)	60 degrees (2)	60 degrees (2)	70 degrees (1)	70 degrees (1)
2.50 to 3.00	70 degrees (2)	70 degrees (2)	70 degrees (2)	60 degrees (2)	60 degrees (2)
3.00 to 4.00	80 degrees (2)	80 degrees (2)	80 degrees (2)	70 degrees(2)	70 degrees(2)
AGAINST-THE-RULE ASTIGMATISM					
Astigmatism (D)	*40 to 50 yo*	*50 to 60 yo*	*60 to 70 yo*	*70 to 80 yo*	*80+ yo*
1.00 to 1.50	60 degrees (1)	50 degrees (1)	40 degrees (1)	40 degrees (1)	30 degrees (1)
1.50 to 2.00	70 degrees (1)	60 degrees (1)	60 degrees (1)	60 degrees (1)	40 degrees (1)
2.00 to 2.50	60 degrees (2)	80 degrees (1)	80 degrees (1)	70 degrees (1)	60 degrees (1)
2.50 to 3.00	70 degrees (2)	70 degrees (2)	70 degrees (2)	60 degrees (2)	60 degrees (2)
3.00 to 4.00	80 degrees (2)	80 degrees (2)	80 degrees (2)	70 degrees (2)	70 degrees (2)

[a]Assumes all cataract incisions are performed temporally and are relatively astigmatically neutral.
(1) denotes one incision; (2) denotes 2 incisions.
Note: When using the nomogram, if age/astigmatism is the dividing point, choose the shortest incision length and choose one incision over 2.

Medicare patients for an additional out-of-pocket fee for LRIs, an Advanced Beneficiary Notice (ABN) should be filed.

My Technique

I prefer to perform LRIs prior to the lens procedure. The cornea is not likely to be as dry and the anterior chamber is stable. The main reason I stopped performing LRIs after the RCS is because I forgot to do the LRI on a few cases that became unexpectedly challenging.

I have designed the "Wallace LRI Kit" with Storz Ophthalmic Instruments, which includes the following:

- A single footplate 600-μm diamond knife
- Mendez axis marker
- 0.12-mm Calibri forceps

The steps of my LRI procedure are as follows:

1. Place the Mendez axis marker on the cornea.
2. Mark the axis with forceps.
3. Turn the Mendez marker so that a primary mark, such as 180 or 30 degrees, is now adjacent to the axis mark.
4. The incision borders are then marked with the forceps; that is 30 degrees on each side for a 60-degree arc.
5. Dry the corneal marks with a Weck-cel sponge (Beaver Visitec).
6. Fixate the globe with the forceps.
7. Advance the knife toward the point of fixation (as recommended by Dr. Douglas Koch) with the knife perpendicular to the corneal surface.
8. Connect the 3 "corneal dots" to complete the corneal arc incision.

Videos of this procedure are available on http://www.YouTube.com; search for Wallace LRI. Also on the YouTube site is a stepwise video of "at home wetlab" methods. The LRI process is one of the few ocular procedures that surgeons can learn at home.

Postoperatively, I routinely prescribe a topical nonsteroidal medication and encourage use of artificial tears. If significant epithelial disruption occurs, I will place an extended-wear soft contact lens, which will be removed the following day.

Key Points About Limbal Relaxing Incisions

- LRIs are not limbal but peripheral corneal incisions placed 1.0 to 1.5 mm anterior to the limbus.
- If keratometry does not correlate with corneal topography, avoid the LRI until measurements can be performed postoperatively.
- Do the LRIs before phaco.
- Low to medium corneal astigmatism can be corrected with a single LRI.
- Femtosecond cataract surgery has tended to validate the benefits of LRIs, but it is undetermined at this time whether surgeons will adopt this new technology. In the meantime, traditional LRI techniques remain an important component to achieve spectacle reduction with refractive lens procedures.

References

1. Verzella F, Calossi A. Multifocal effect of against-the-rule myopic astigmatism in pseudophakic eyes. *J Refract Corneal Surg.* 1993;9(58-61.
2. Sawusch M, Guyton D. Optimal astigmatism to enhance depth of focus after cataract surgery. *Ophthalmology.* 1991;98:1025-1029.
3. Wallace RB. On-axis cataract incisions: where is the axis? In: *1995 ASCRS Symposium of Cataract, IOL and Refractive Surgery Best Papers of Sessions.* Fairfax, VA: ASCRS; 1995:67-72.
4. Wallace RB. Reducing astigmatism. In: Wallace RB, ed. *Refractive Cataract Surgery and Multifocal IOLs.* Thorofare, NJ: SLACK Incorporated; 2001:167-172.

5

Enhancement of Patients With Prior Limbal Relaxing Incisions

David R. Hardten, MD and Molly McDonald, OD

The precision of refractive outcomes after lens surgery has greatly improved in the past few decades. Our ability to control astigmatism is better with small-incision cataract surgery compared with extracapsular cataract surgery, where residual astigmatism greater than 1.00 diopters (D) was common.[1-3] Nonetheless, it is not always possible to exactly achieve the desired refractive result with lens surgery alone—the patient may have pre-existing corneal astigmatism, and even with the most meticulous preoperative measurements and calculations, natural anatomic variability can lead to residual refractive error. Such refractive error may include myopia, hyperopia, and/or astigmatism.

Although current methods to reduce pre-existing astigmatism, such as limbal relaxing incisions (LRIs) or toric intraocular lenses (IOLs), can effectively reduce corneal astigmatism at the time of cataract surgery, the patient may still have postoperative residual spherical or astigmatic refractive error that evokes symptoms worthy of further surgical correction. The management of this residual refractive error may best be addressed, in most cases, through laser vision correction. Although further LRIs or other incisional techniques, IOL exchange, or rotation of a toric IOL are additional options, these are not, in our experience, as effective as excimer surgery.

In general, undercorrections are typically better tolerated than overcorrections, and although additional surgery may be performed for residual refractive error, it should be remembered that the simplest form of management is the use of spectacles or contact lenses. Further surgical intervention should be undertaken only after a thorough discussion of the available options, risks, and benefits has been offered to the patient.

Especially when contemplating a second intraocular surgery, consideration and discussion must take place in regard to the potential for cystoid macular edema, endothelial cell loss, retinal detachment, and increased intraocular inflammation. For these reasons, an intraocular technique is not utilized as commonly as laser vision correction.

In our experience, the most precise method to correct residual ametropia is laser vision correction. When planned in advance, laser vision correction has been termed *bioptics*, as some patients may require the need for 2 different surgeries to achieve the desired result.[4,5] The precision of the excimer laser is unparalleled in its ability to achieve targeted refractive outcomes. Use of the excimer laser for the treatment of myopia, hyperopia, and astigmatism has made great strides over the past 20 years, and it is now well established. It has been clearly demonstrated that

Nichamin LD.
Limbal Relaxing Incisions: A Practical Guide (pp 85-91).

photorefractive keratectomy (PRK) and laser in situ keratomileusis (LASIK) are predictable and effective means of correcting various types and degrees of ametropia, including astigmatism.[6-17]

Techniques

When a stable refractive error is confirmed by careful refraction, additional parameters pertinent to laser vision correction are obtained. These may include wavefront, topography, keratometry, and pachymetry measurements. Ideally, these measurements are obtained prior to the primary lens surgery to determine whether a laser correcting procedure, if needed, is possible or safe following the implant procedure. Refractive stability will typically occur by 1-month postoperatively with small-incision cataract surgery, particularly when an overlapping anterior capsulorrhexis is achieved with a modern-style IOL, even when LRIs have been performed. Despite this stability, we typically wait 3 months after lens surgery before performing a laser vision correction enhancement. At that time, there is likely no concern for wound dehiscence with further surgery, especially with well-constructed, self-sealing incisions.

Patient Selections

Pachymetry measurements are also important, especially if considering LASIK. We typically will use PRK after a patient has had LRIs to avoid any crossing of the incisions with the LASIK flap, but if the incisions are peripheral enough where the flap will not cross the LRI, then LASIK is a reasonable option. Topography helps in identifying the risk factors for postoperative ectasia and other forms of irregular astigmatism. Because the patient has had cataract incisions and LRIs, some amount of irregular astigmatism is typical.

Next, a thorough general ophthalmic examination should be performed. Treatment of blepharitis with lid hygiene, and correction of lid problems, such as entropion or ectropion, should be considered prior to keratorefractive surgery to reduce issues with dry eye and healing. A careful slit-lamp examination will help to identify keratoconjunctivitis sicca, anterior basement membrane dystrophy (ABMD), corneal neovascularization, endothelial disease, and the clarity of the posterior capsule—all important issues to be considered prior to laser vision surgery.

In particular, significant preoperative dry eye should be treated aggressively prior to laser surgery with artificial tears, ointments, topical cyclosporine, heating treatments of the lids, and/or punctal plugs. In the presence of ABMD, a surface ablation is preferred to avoid epithelial sloughing, which increases the risk of epithelial ingrowth. Corneal neovascularization may be problematic, as it can lead to intraoperative bleeding that may interfere with the ablation or reduce flap adherence in LASIK, thus making PRK preferable in such cases. Posterior capsular opacification may interfere with accurate refractions and wavefront aberrometry. Hence, where indicated, neodymium yttrium-aluminum-garnet (Nd:YAG) capsulotomy should be performed prior to the enhancement.

Finally, a careful fundus examination should be performed to exclude the presence of cystoid macular edema, which can also affect refractive error, in addition to best-corrected visual acuity.

Treatment

Some patients will prefer bilateral simultaneous laser surgery if both eyes require enhancements. This avoids anisometropia, the inconvenience and stress of returning for 2 procedures, and the recovery protocol and visits required if the surgeries are performed at 2 separate times. However, especially in surface laser enhancement, where visual recovery is slower than with a

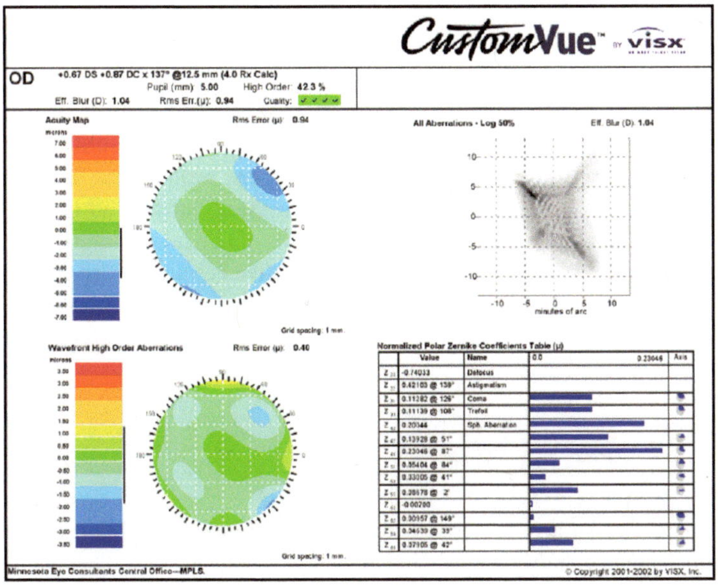

Figure 5-1. Wavefront of a patient with residual astigmatism after cataract surgery and IOL implantation. The patient also has mild hyperopia in addition to the astigmatism, which makes laser vision correction ideal for managing both the spherical and astigmatic components. This patient had final uncorrected vision at 3 months after PRK enhancement.

lamellar procedure, some patients will opt for unilateral treatment. The refractive errors are typically relatively small, and unilateral treatment allows for functional vision in the nonoperated eye during the recovery period.

Residual astigmatism is often accompanied by some degree of spherical error, and laser vision correction not only affords the opportunity to reduce or eliminate cylinder but also problematic myopia or hyperopia. It is widely appreciated that LASIK provides a quicker visual recovery than surface ablation (eg, PRK, laser epithelial keratomileusis, epi-LASIK); hence, when possible, most patients will prefer this approach. However, in certain cases, a surface procedure may be safer, particularly in the cataract-aged population. Conditions such as ABMD, thin corneas, and suspicious topographic patterns are not uncommon and are typically best suited for a surface ablation treatment.

Custom Treatments

Lower-order corrections are typically most important following IOL surgery, and laser vision correction is quite accurate for these typically nominal errors. Still, wavefront analyzers for custom laser refractive procedures can be used to treat higher-order aberrations that negatively impact the optics of the visual system. By applying wavefront analysis, coma, trefoil, spherical aberration, or other higher-order aberrations can be targeted and reduced in many patients where they may be visually significant (WaveScan; Abbott Medical Optics). Still, because of the small corrections and difficulty with obtaining wavefront measurements in IOL patients, especially those with a multifocal IOL, standard treatments are also very successful.

One advantage of using custom PRK is that astigmatic targeting is improved with iris registration and pupil centroid shift, which is available through wavefront aberrometry measurements (Figure 5-1). If the patient underwent multifocal IOL implantation, especially using a refractive IOL such as the ReZoom (Abbott Medical Optics Inc) or the Array (Abbott Medical Optics Inc), the wavefront measurements may be unreliable. In diffractive IOLs, such as the Tecnis multifocal (Abbott Medical Optics Inc) or the ReStor (Alcon Surgical), a reliable wavefront measurement is often obtainable, especially if the anterior capsulorrhexis is not too small. Typically, a 4.5- to 5.5-mm anterior capsulorrhexis will allow capture of 5 mm of information from the wavefront if it is well centered and there is no posterior capsular opacity. It is also important that the patient's uncorrected visual acuity correlates with his or her refraction, especially when managing the multifocal IOL patient. Care should be taken not to refract the near zones of the IOLs. For example, a red flag should go up if refraction indicates the need for an ablation of -2.00 D for a patient whose visual acuity is 20/40 uncorrected at distance. In addition, especially for astigmatic errors, a match between the topographic astigmatism and the refracted and wavefront astigmatism should verify that the axis of treatment and amounts are similar. Some degree of irregular astigmatism may be seen in patients who have had prior LRIs, as the match is not always perfect, but a trend toward agreement is important. Surface PRK in patients with moderate amounts of irregular astigmatism is quite successful.[18] Based on the study by Van Gelder et al,[19] refractive results in flap-based and PRK-based procedures are comparable in mild-to-moderate myopia patients, but flap-based procedures are better in high myopia patients[19] (which is typically not an issue in postcataract patients).

Procedure

When performing PRK, we generally remove the epithelium to expose Bowman's layer, using dilute (20% to 70%) alcohol, although mechanical epithelial removal is also possible.[20-23] Care should be taken to remove all the epithelium within the ablation zone because any residual epithelial cells will create small areas of irregularity and may affect the smoothness of the ablation surface. Alcohol removal is typically faster and easier for the occasional PRK surgeon to learn and use. It may also have a slightly quicker recovery period.

We typically place 70% alcohol on a thin, nonfragmenting cellulose dot and squeeze out most of the fluid to where the dot is only slightly moist. We then paint the epithelium with alcohol for 10 to 20 seconds, taking care not to damage the limbal stem cells. The excess alcohol evaporates from the surface within 2 to 3 seconds. The loosened epithelium is removed using another dry sponge or a PRK spatula. Despite the loss of keratocytes and inflammation in the stroma when alcohol is used, most patients do well clinically.[21]

When the epithelium is completely removed, corneal hydration is checked to make sure that it is not excessively moist or dry. Typically, no adjustment of hydration is needed if the epithelial removal has been relatively rapid. The patient is asked to maintain his or her gaze on the fixation target, the eye tracker and iris registration are engaged, and the laser energy is centered on the pupil. Laser treatment should proceed at this point, ensuring that the patient maintains proper fixation. The corneal hydration status should be monitored carefully to prevent excessive dehydration or extra fluid collection in the stromal tissue, which can affect the refractive outcome.

Transepithelial ablation with the excimer laser is sometimes performed, although this practice is not as common because the epithelial thickness varies in different patients, especially with relaxing incisions that are more central.

Following laser treatment, mitomycin C (MMC) in a concentration ranging from 0.1 to 0.2 mg/mL (0.01% to 0.02%) may be used to reduce the potential for the development of haze.[24-26] The amount of time that the MMC is used is typically shorter (15 to 30 seconds) for these ablations, as the amount of correction is relatively small, yet longer times (up to 2 minutes) may be considered if the PRK zone crosses the relaxing incisions. A bandage contact lens is placed over the eye. The patient is given topical steroids, antibiotics, and nonsteroidal anti-inflammatory eye drops. If a high correction is performed, the patient may also be instructed to begin taking 1 g of vitamin C daily, which has been shown to inhibit haze formation.[27,28] Artificial tears should be used copiously to maintain proper hydration of the bandage contact lens and aid in wound healing.

Postoperative Management

The patient should return for follow-up care on postoperative day 1 for an examination of the newly forming epithelial surface underneath the bandage contact lens. This examination can be accomplished without removal of the lens, so as not to interrupt the leading edge of the epithelium.

The patient is seen next at approximately postoperative day 4 or 5 for removal of the bandage contact lens after the epithelium has healed completely. We typically remove the bandage contact lens with a dull forceps or cotton tip applicator to limit epithelial disruption. After removal of the bandage contact lens, the patient begins using a hyperosmotic ophthalmic ointment (eg, sodium chloride 5%) at bedtime.

Postoperative medications vary, particularly in accordance with the use of steroids. Some physicians prefer to limit topical steroidal use to 2 weeks, whereas others may elect to keep their patients on steroidal medications for 2 to 3 months postoperatively.

Photorefractive keratectomy and LASIK have been shown to produce predictable and effective treatment of ametropia, including astigmatism.[6-17] In fact, the excimer laser procedure has essentially replaced incisional astigmatic keratotomy for the correction of astigmatism in many settings, except in combination with IOL surgery. Proper attention to surgical details, as well as preoperative and postoperative management, will continue to provide safe and reliable astigmatic corrections. Complications from LASIK and PRK are unusual, and if managed appropriately, a minimal incidence of loss of best-corrected visual acuity exists.

Complications

Although complications are uncommon in using PRK after LRIs, when LASIK has been used in patients with radial incisions, intraoperative incision opening and wound dehiscence, irregular apposition of the flap to the stromal bed, stromal opacities, epithelial defects, decentered ablations, epithelial ingrowth, corneal haze, and corneal ectasia may occur.[29-35] However, such problems are not typically encountered following prior LRIs.

The occurrence of general complications following laser enhancement surgery is, however, possible and must be shared with the patient through informed consent. These complications would include over- and undercorrection, delayed healing, increased dry eye, scarring, irregular astigmatism, and infection. All of these complications are, fortunately, rare events.

Conclusion

Although most patients will achieve the refractive goal after cataract surgery with relaxing incisions, it is important to be prepared for the patient with residual refractive error. Addressing this residual refractive error is important to achieve the high level of patients' expectations. Careful planning of the enhancement surgery includes waiting for the refractive error to become stable, managing posterior capsular opacity, and other intraocular and surface problems that may be contributing to poor best-corrected vision, as well as determining that the refractive error is characterized in a similar manner among the refraction, topography, and wavefront analysis. Our preferred method for the management of residual refractive error in a patient who has undergone prior LRIs is to perform PRK with MMC using wavefront analysis. With this approach, most patients can achieve excellent uncorrected visual acuity.

References

1. Gills JP. Treating astigmatism at the time of cataract surgery. *Curr Opin Ophthalmol.* 2002;13(1):2-6.
2. Nichamin LD. Treating astigmatism at the time of cataract surgery. *Curr Opin Ophthalmol.* 2003;14(1):35-38.
3. Nichamin LD. Astigmatism management for modern phaco surgery. *Int Ophthalmol Clin.* 2003;43(3):53-63.
4. Chayet AS, Magallanes R, Montes M, Chavez S, Robledo N. Laser in situ keratomileusis for simple myopic, mixed, and simple hyperopic astigmatism. *J Refract Surg.* 1998;14(2 Suppl):S175-S176.
5. Zaldivar R, Davidorf JM, Oscherow S, Ricur G, Piezzi V. Combined posterior chamber phakic intraocular lens and laser in situ keratomileusis: bioptics for extreme myopia. *J Refract Surg.* 1999;15(3):299-308.
6. Nichamin LD. Expanding the role of bioptics to the pseudophakic patient. *J Cataract Refract Surg.* 2001;27(9):1343-1344.
7. Dausch D, Klein R, Landesz M, Schroder E. Photorefractive keratectomy to correct astigmatism with myopia or hyperopia. *J Cataract Refract Surg.* 1994;20(Suppl):252-257.
8. Davidorf JM, Zaldivar R, Oscherow S. Results and complications of laser in situ keratomileusis by experienced surgeons. *J Refract Surg.* 1998;14(2):114-122.
9. Ditzen K, Huschka H, Pieger S. Laser in situ keratomileusis for hyperopia. *J Cataract Refract Surg.* 1998;24(1):42-47.
10. Gartry DS, Kerr Muir MG, Marshall J. Excimer laser photorefractive keratectomy. 18-month follow-up. *Ophthalmology.* 1992;99(8):1209-1219.
11. Ibrahim O. Laser in situ keratomileusis for hyperopia and hyperopic astigmatism. *J Refract Surg.* 1998;14(2 Suppl):S179-S182.
12. Jabbur NS, Kraff C. Wavefront-guided laser in situ keratomileusis using the WaveScan system for correction of low to moderate myopia with astigmatism: 6-month results in 277 eyes. *J Cataract Refract Surg.* 2005;31(8):1493-1501.
13. Knorz MC, Liermann A, Jendritza B, Hugger P. LASIK for hyperopia and hyperopic astigmatism¾results of a pilot study. *Semin Ophthalmol.* 1998;13(2):83-87.
14. Lee JS, Oum BS, Lee BJ, Lee SH. Photorefractive keratectomy for astigmatism greater than -2.00 diopters in eyes with low, high, or extreme myopia. *J Cataract Refract Surg.* 1998;24(11):1456-1463.
15. Sher NA, Chen V, Bowers RA, et al. The use of the 193-nm excimer laser for myopic photorefractive keratectomy in sighted eyes: a multicenter study. *Arch Ophthalmol.* 1991;109(11):1525-1530.
16. Partal AE, Manche EE. CustomVue laser in situ keratomileusis for myopia and myopic astigmatism using the Visx S4 excimer laser: efficacy, predictability, and safety. *J Cataract Refract Surg.* 2006;32(3):475-479.
17. Pallikaris IG, Siganos DS. Excimer laser in situ keratomileusis and photorefractive keratectomy for correction of high myopia. *J Refract Corneal Surg.* 1994;10(5):498-510.
18. Hardten DR, Lindstrom RL, Fogal BJ. *Wavefront excimer laser surface ablation for significant levels of coma and trefoil.* Paper presented at: the American Society of Cataract and Refractive Surgery Symposium on Cataract, IOL, and Refractive Surgery; April 27-May 2, 2007; San Diego, CA.
19. Van Gelder RN, Steger-May K, Yang SH, Rattanatam T, Pepose JS. Comparison of photorefractive keratectomy, astigmatic PRK, laser in situ keratomileusis, and astigmatic LASIK in the treatment of myopia. *J Cataract Refract Surg.* 2002;28(3):462-476.
20. Abad JC, An B, Power WJ, Foster CS, Azar DT, Talamo JH. A prospective evaluation of alcohol-assisted versus mechanical epithelial removal before photorefractive keratectomy. *Ophthalmology.* 1997;104(10):1566-1574.
21. Agrawal VB, Hanuch OE, Bassage S, Aquavella JV. Alcohol versus mechanical epithelial debridement: effect on underlying cornea before excimer laser surgery. *J Cataract Refract Surg.* 1997;23(8):1153-1159.
22. Stein HA, Stein RM, Price C, Salim GA. Alcohol removal of the epithelium for excimer laser ablation: outcomes analysis. *J Cataract Refract Surg.* 1997;23(8):1160-1163.
23. Ghoreishi M, Attarzadeh H, Tavakoli M, et al. Alcohol-assisted versus mechanical epithelium removal in photorefractive keratectomy. *J Ophthalmic Vis Res.* 2010;5(4):223-227.
24. Majmudar PA, Forstot SL, Dennis RF, et al. Topical mitomycin-C for subepithelial fibrosis after refractive corneal surgery. *Ophthalmology.* 2000;107(1):89-94.
25. Vigo L, Scandola E, Carones F. Scraping and mitomycin C to treat haze and regression after photorefractive keratectomy for myopia. *J Refract Surg.* 2003;19(4):449-454.
26. Carones F, Vigo L, Scandola E, Vacchini L. Evaluation of prophylactic of mitomycin-C to inhibit haze formation after photorefractive keratectomy. *J Cataract Refract Surg.* 2002;28(12):2088-2095.
27. Stojanovic A, Ringvold A, Nitter T. Ascorbate prophylaxis for corneal haze after photorefractive keratectomy. *J Refract Surg.* 2003;19(3):338-343.
28. Hayes S, Cafaro TA, Boguslawska PJ, et al. The effect of vitamin C deficiency and chronic ultraviolet-B exposure on corneal ultrastructure: a preliminary investigation. *Mol Vis.* 2011;17:3107-3115.
29. Oral D, Awwad ST, Seward MS, Bowman RW, McCulley JP, Cavanagh HD. Hyperopic laser in situ keratomileusis in eyes with previous radial keratotomy. *J Cataract Refract Surg.* 2005;31(8):1561-1568.

30. Francesconi CM, Nose RA, Nose W. Hyperopic laser-assisted in situ keratomileusis for radial keratotomy induced hyperopia. *Ophthalmology.* 2002;109(3):602-605.
31. Agarwal A, Agarwal A, Agarwal T, Bagmar A, Agarwal S. Laser in situ keratomileusis for residual myopia after radial keratotomy and photorefractive keratectomy. *J Cataract Refract Surg.* 2001;27(6):901-906.
32. Attia WH, Alió JL, Artola A, Muñoz G, Shalaby AM. Laser in situ keratomileusis for undercorrection and overcorrection after radial keratotomy. *J Cataract Refract Surg.* 2001;27(2):267-272.
33. Shah SB, Lingua RW, Kim CH, Peters NT. Laser in situ keratomileusis to correct residual myopia and astigmatism after radial keratotomy. *J Cataract Refract Surg.* 2000;26(8):1152-1157.
34. Clausse MA, Boutros G, Khanjian G, Wagner C, Garabet AL. A retrospective study of laser in situ keratomileusis after radial keratotomy. *J Refract Surg.* 2001;17(2 Suppl):S200-S201.
35. Muñoz G, Montés-Micó R, Albarrán-Diego C, Alió JL. Keratectasia after bilateral laser in situ keratomileusis in a patient with previous radial and astigmatic keratotomy. *J Cataract Refract Surg.* 2005;31(2):441-445.

6

Limbal Relaxing Incision Complications

Parag D. Parekh, MD, MPA

"Chance favors the prepared mind." ~Louis Pasteur

There is but one way to avoid complications—perform no surgery and there will be no complications. We all should study complications—how and why they occur, what can be done to minimize risk, and what can be done when they inevitably occur.

In the case of an elective refractive procedure, the level of safety and predictability that we pursue is of paramount importance. This chapter will provide an overview of limbal relaxing incision (LRI)-related complications, both prevention and management.

Vision-Threatening Complications

Perforation

Microperforation is a small, full-thickness perforation of the cornea and is suspected when aqueous appears on the corneal surface while performing a relaxing incision. Unlike the "micro" perforations that occur in conjunction with radial keratotomy (RK), most perforations that occur with transverse or circum-parallel astigmatic incisions will not self-seal.

As soon as excess fluid is noted, the surgeon must immediately differentiate between simple surface fluid that typically originates from the conjunctival fornix and appears as the eye is depressed during the procedure versus actual aqueous—indicating entry into the anterior chamber. In either case, one should *stop* and assess the situation. In the case of pooling surface fluid, the incision may be continued after drying of the fornices with a sponge. If a full-thickness perforation has occurred, in most cases it is best to defer completion of the incision until after both the corneal thickness and instrument status has been checked and the etiology of the perforation has been determined. The two most common causes of a perforation include unrecognized peripheral corneal thinning or pathology or faulty instrumentation; after many sterilization cycles, the micrometer mechanism in the knife may slip and a faulty depth setting may be present.

Nichamin LD.
Limbal Relaxing Incisions: A Practical Guide (pp 93-97).

In the event of a perforation, the surgeon should further assess the situation and consider the following:

- Check the anterior chamber depth—is it still formed?
- Confirm that the iris and other anterior segment structures are unaffected.
- Consider the intraocular pressure—was the globe hyperinflated?
- Recheck the corneal thickness in the area of the intended incision.
- Recheck the intended blade depth.
- Does the blade depth indicator need to be recalibrated?
- Did hand position or patient anatomy (prominent brow) contribute?
- Was the cornea excessively dehydrated?

When the cause of perforation is addressed, in some cases it may be possible to complete the LRI; after decreasing its depth setting, the blade may be reinserted into the partial incision, and the cut completed to its intended arc length. More frequently, however, the incision must be abandoned, and it must be sealed if it is leaky. Again, unlike RK, astigmatic incisions have a marked proclivity for leakage and typically require suturing, even to allow completion of the cataract and implant procedure.

A longer macroperforation is a more serious complication and mandates that the LRI surgery be aborted. Nylon 10-0 sutures are typically placed perpendicular to the incision to seal the perforation. The surgeon must specifically confirm that the iris is not incarcerated into the perforation. In addition, for those surgeons who perform LRI immediately prior to cataract surgery, the integrity of the anterior capsule should be confirmed.

Depending on the extent of the macroperforation and the stability and healing of the corneal incision, sutures can typically be removed in approximately 8 weeks postoperatively, often in a titrated fashion. Alternatively, if the postoperative refractive result is acceptable, the sutures may be left intact. Following suture removal and documentation of a stable refraction and corneal topography, additional corneal surgery may be offered, depending on the clinical circumstances and the patient's subjective status. Laser vision correction, rather than additional incisional surgery, may be a preferable postoperative enhancement strategy.

Infection

As always, a surgical incision can lead to infection. Fortunately, infectious keratitis rarely occurs after LRI, with the infiltrate located within or adjacent to the incision. Improper aseptic technique may be the causative factor, along with pre-existing external disease. Most physicians use both pre- and postoperative topical antibiotics (off-label use) for infection prophylaxis, in addition to use of a preoperative iodine solution during the preoperative surgical preparation and draping. Epithelial defects and bandage contact lenses may increase the incidence of infection.

I typically follow the usual infectious keratitis protocol for this complication, and I would suggest immediate culturing. As with all corneal infections, sequelae can include corneal scarring, thinning, irregular astigmatism, and, rarely, perforation and endophthalmitis. Sterile infiltrates are also possible, and patients with rheumatoid disease, severe dry eye, and certain long-term topical medications may be particularly predisposed.[1,2]

Endophthalmitis

Post-LRI endophthalmitis has been rarely reported,[3] but it can be a devastating complication. The route of pathogen entry could be via mircoperforation, macroperforation, or LRI-related infectious keratitis.

As with any infection, rapid diagnosis and treatment is vital to preserving postoperative visual function. As with cataract surgery, in general, pre-existing external disease should be addressed and controlled prior to surgical intervention.

Anesthesia-Related Complications

Although it is not the focus of this text, the surgeon should keep in mind the potential challenges of anesthesia. Most LRI surgery is performed with topical anesthesia, where patient discomfort, movement, and lid squeezing has the potential to lead to an imprecise incision. Surgery performed with retrobulbar anesthesia risks globe perforation and retrobulbar hemorrhage,[4] but it may afford the surgeon, particularly the novice surgeon, more intraoperative control.

Side Effects and Nonvision-Threatening Complications

Pain, Foreign Body Sensation, and Dry Eye

Patients may experience mild discomfort after surgery, when the analgesia provided by the topical or retrobulbar anesthesia subsides. Rarely, this can persist beyond a few hours, or even 1 to 2 days. Frequent lubricants and the use of a topical nonsteroidal medication can greatly reduce such symptoms.

Some patients may demonstrate punctate epithelial staining postoperatively, either from excessive corneal dehydration during surgery or potentially due to decreased corneal sensation, as the LRI severs local corneal nerves. Correcting larger amounts of astigmatism necessitates a longer LRI, which in turn severs more nerves, leaving a larger amount of the cornea neurotrophic. Patients with decreased corneal sensation prior to surgery, such as diabetics and those with a history of herpetic keratitis, exposure keratopathy, or other neurotrophic pathology, may be at higher risk. Furthermore, autoimmune and connective tissue diseases, such as rheumatoid arthritis, systemic lupus erythematosus, ankylosing spondylitis, psoriatic arthritis, Sjögren's syndrome, Wegener's granulomatosis, relapsing polychondritis, polyarteritis nodosa, or atopia, may alter the corneal healing response.[5] Rarely, a nonhealing defect or neurotrophic ulcer may result.[6] Any ocular surface defect in the epithelium or tear film can impact visual acuity and result in a long-term reduction in postoperative visual acuity.

Of note, the cataract incision itself can lead to decreased corneal sensation,[7] and the addition of an LRI, especially a long one, may exacerbate this type of problem.[8]

Epithelial Defect

Epithelial defects are typically mild after LRIs and can result from underlying epithelial basement membrane dystrophy (EBMD), as well as inadequate corneal surface lubrication during incision creation or a defective LRI instrument (eg, dull blade, irregular footplate). Healing may be delayed due to the decreased corneal sensation mentioned previously. Recurrent corneal erosions can also occur as a consequence of the initial epithelial defect, especially in the context of EBMD.

An epithelial defect can lead to temporary blurred vision, photophobia, glare, monocular diplopia, and, rarely, corneal scarring; therefore, the surgeon must work to bring about resolution of the defect as quickly as possible.

Bandage contact lenses, copious topical lubrication, warm compresses, doxycycline, punctal plugs, pressure patching, and serum tears can all help to resolve a surface defect. In addition, optimization of the ocular surface with these measures preoperatively may also help to decrease the incidence of dry eye, foreign body sensation, and epithelial defects postoperatively.

Fluctuating Refraction

In the first few days after surgery, diffuse corneal edema related to cataract surgery and localized edema related to the LRI normally resolve without issue. Refractive stability, related to both effective lens position and capsular contraction, as well as corneal stability of the LRI, is ordinarily achieved within a few weeks. The latter can be confirmed with keratometry readings and topography. The proper use of anti-inflammatories and surface lubrication may help in hastening refractive stabilization.

Irregular Noncurvilinear Incision

As other authors have noted throughout this book, the LRI is ideally made as a single, smooth, gently curved, arcuate incision, with the LRI blade held perpendicular to the corneal surface. Many factors can lead to deviations from this ideal.

Patient-related issues, such as sudden movement or difficult positioning, can cause irregular incisions or an LRI that is too long or too short. Prior preparation and anticipating potential difficulty is essential. The surgeon must pay special attention to the patient's head position, as well as his or her own hand position in all cases, but especially for the patient with a deep set eye or prominent brow. The surgeon should take care to ensure the patient's comfort, and give the patient a good fixation target for this delicate and precise part of the surgery. In addition, a gentle verbal reminder to hold steady during the LRI can help prevent sudden head and eye movement. If the incision is too long, too short, too shallow, wanders off the intended track, or is placed at a nonperpendicular angle, a resultant over- or undercorrection may occur. Very rarely, irregular astigmatism may be induced, especially if the incision veers centrally toward the visual axis.

Surgical technique, including improper hand movement or poor patient exposure, may lead to an irregular, noncurvilinear incision. An important surgical pearl is to take a moment to stabilize one's hands and fingers on the patient—gently placing one's fingers on the surgical drape above the patient's brow, nose, or cheek in an ergonomic position prior to commencing the incision—and confirm adequate support. Fortunately, in most cases, LRIs are very forgiving—a mildly irregular or serpentine incision will typically have little detrimental effect on the visual outcome.

Overcorrection or Undercorrection

An important source of error is the placement of LRIs in the incorrect location. Avoiding this problem begins with having a clear and documented surgical plan prior to entering the operating room and the proper marking of the patient preoperatively. Many studies indicate that significant cyclorotation can occur while the patient is in the supine position on the operating table. Therefore, one's orientation, or reference points, might not be where the surgeon thinks they are, leading to misplacement of the LRI, off of the true steep meridian .

As such, many surgeons believe that it is important for the patient to be marked in an upright position, sitting on a chair or bed, fixating on a distance target, with the head in a neutral position. In addition, it may be helpful to place several marks (eg, dots at 90 and 180 degrees), in the event that some of the marks fade during the preoperative preparation. If the surgeon performs the LRI at the conclusion of cataract surgery and finds that the marks are fading at any point, the reinforcement of these limbal landmarks should be undertaken to maintain proper orientation and placement of the relaxing incisions.

A common error is to confuse the steep and the flat axis. A surgeon can easily mistake the astigmatic meridian for the axis or mistake a plus cylinder notation for a minus cylinder notation and place the LRI 90 degrees away from where it should be, often leading to a doubling of the refractive cylinder. As a reminder, the LRI incisions should be placed on the steep meridian, which equates to the plus cylinder axis.

In the event of undercorrection, the LRI incision can be extended postoperatively, after refractive stability is achieved. In the event of overcorrection and flipping of the astigmatic axis, the LRI wound can be opened and the edges of the incision can be reapproximated with 10-0 nylon sutures after the epithelial plug, if present, is removed. One to 2 months later, the nylon sutures can be removed, and when the corneal topography and refraction are stable, the surgeon may consider placing another LRI to neutralize the astigmatism.

In this situation, a nonincisional enhancement modality, such as an excimer laser-based treatment—laser in situ keratomileusis or photorefractive keratectomy—may be considered to correct both the residual astigmatism and any remaining spherical errors. Other modalities, including intraoperative keratoscopy or wavefront aberrometry can also help to prevent and treat these types of complications.

Conclusion

LRI is characteristically a safe and effective way to manage astigmatism, but complications are possible. The surgeon should strive to understand the possible complications, take steps to prevent them, and know how to manage them when they (inevitably) occur.

References

1. Lin JC, Rapuano CJ, Laibson PR, Eagle RC Jr, Cohen EJ. Corneal melting associated with use of topical nonsteroidal anti-inflammatory drugs after ocular surgery. *Arch Ophthalmol.* 2000;118(8):1129-1132.
2. Flach AJ. Corneal melts associated with topically applied nonsteroidal anti-inflammatory drugs. *Trans Am Ophthalmol Soc.* 2001;99:205-210.
3. Haripriya A, Syeda T. A case of endophthalmitis associated with limbal relaxing incision. *Indian J Ophthalmol.* 2012;60(3):223-225.
4. Ramsay RC, Knobloch WH. Ocular perforation following retrobulbar anesthesia for retinal detachment surgery. *Am J Ophthalmol.* 1978;86(1):61-64.
5. Robin JB, Dugel R, Robin SB. Immunologic disorders of the cornea and conjunctiva. In: Kaufman HE, Barron BA, McDonald MB, eds, *The Cornea.* Boston, MA, Butterworth-Heinemann, 1998; 551-595.
6. Moon S-W, Yeom D-J, Chung S-H. Neurotrophic corneal ulcer development following cataract surgery with a limbal relaxing incision. *Korean J Ophthalmol.* 2011;25(3):210-213.
7. Kohlhass, M. Corneal sensation after cataract and refractive surgery. *J Cataract Refract Surg.* 1998;24(1):1399-1409.
8. Donnenfeld ED, Holland EJ, Nichamin LD, et al. *A multicenter evaluation of the effects of cataract extraction and limbal relaxing incisions on corneal sensation.* Poster (PO314) presented at: the American Academy of Ophthalmology Annual Meeting; October 24, 2011; Orlando, FL.

7

Femtosecond Laser Limbal Relaxing Incisions

Eric D. Donnenfeld, MD; Allon Barsam, MD, MA, FRCOphth; and An Vo, MD

Cataract surgery is one of the most commonly performed procedures worldwide and has, in large part, become a refractive procedure in which patients have increasingly high expectations for both functional visual improvement as well as spectacle independence.[1,2]

Management of astigmatism, in particular, may be the most important aspect in the quest to maximizing surgical outcomes, as optimal postoperative uncorrected visual acuity has become the main measure of success for patients undergoing refractive cataract surgery. Astigmatism decreases visual acuity through meridional blur, in which one axis of the cornea is steeper than the other, causing distortion of the visual image. Residual astigmatism after cataract surgery of 0.50 diopters (D) or less may result in glare, symptomatic blur, ghosting, and halos.[3] As a result, greater emphasis has been placed on treating corneal astigmatism at the time of cataract surgery with limbal relaxing incisions (LRIs). A recent study of 4540 eyes of 2415 patients showed that corneal astigmatism is present in the majority of patients undergoing cataract surgery, with at least 1.50 D measured in 22.2% of study eyes.[4] Approximately 38% of eyes undergoing cataract surgery have at least 1.00 D of pre-existing corneal astigmatism, and 72% of patients have 0.50 D or more.[5]

Management of astigmatism is important, regardless of the intraocular lens (IOL) that is used. Patients implanted with presbyopia-correcting IOLs, however, are significantly more sensitive to even minor refractive error than those implanted with conventional monofocal IOLs. Refractive IOL surgeons must be willing and able to treat small amounts of postoperative astigmatism to achieve happy postoperative patients.

Astigmatic incisions are corneal incisions that are used to relax and flatten the steep meridian of regular corneal astigmatism while steepening the opposing flat meridian. The procedure reduces corneal tension and allows the cornea to heal into a more spherical shape. Incisions placed adjacent to the limbus are referred to as LRIs, and incisions placed central to the limbus and closer to the visual axis have historically been termed *astigmatic keratotomy* (AK). Because there are several advantages of LRIs over AK, the former are now performed more frequently. These advantages include a reduced tendency to cause axial shift, less irregular astigmatism, a 1:1 coupling ratio, a decreased chance of visually significant scarring, and a reduced likelihood of perforation.

Unfortunately, many cataract surgeons are uncomfortable performing manual incisional astigmatic surgery. In a survey of 233 surgeons, only 73 routinely performed LRIs.[6] Several different options for treating astigmatism exist, including excimer laser photoablation, toric IOL

Nichamin LD.
Limbal Relaxing Incisions: A Practical Guide (pp 99-108).

implantation, and conductive keratoplasty. Each of these options has their respective advantages and shortcomings and may have variable accessibility to cataract surgeons and their patients.

The Limbal Relaxing Incision Procedure

When the required location of the incision has been ascertained, the incision length and depth are determined by the surgeon. Sometimes, a nomogram may be consulted. There are a number of LRI nomograms for correcting varying amounts of cylinder, and many studies evaluating LRIs have been performed.[7-20] In one study that assessed the effectiveness of LRIs, a 60% average reduction of cylinder was noted,[21] with 79% of patients corrected to less than 1.00 D of cylinder and 59% corrected to less than 0.50 D. The 60% reduction in astigmatism compares favorably with the results achieved using toric IOLs, which resulted in a mean 58.4% reduction in cylinder.[22]

Some LRI nomograms are adjusted for age and cylinder axis, making them more detailed and complex, which may give the impression that the procedure is extremely precise and unforgiving. In our opinion, however, this simply is not the case. The LRI procedure has numerous areas for error, and the many variables that are associated with how the incision is performed can each contribute to inconsistency. The incision itself, if performed manually, is only as precise as the surgeon making the incision and the accuracy of the blade. Any of these errors can result in suboptimal visual acuity.

In addition, the phacoemulsification incision and its surgically induced astigmatism (SIA) must be factored into the preoperative astigmatic plan. Using vector analysis, the surgeon should determine the proper meridian in which to place the astigmatic relaxing incisions. All of these factors can be calculated online at http://www.LRIcalculator.com (Abbott Medical Optics Inc [Figure 7-1]). This online LRI calculator uses vector analysis to calculate where to make the LRI incisions based on the patient's preoperative keratometry and the surgeon's induced astigmatism. The LRI calculator also uses the Donnenfeld and Nichamin nomograms and provides a visual map of the axis and length of the incisions that are to be performed.[23,24] A printout of the LRI calculator can be brought to the operating room and used as a guide when marking the cornea and performing LRIs.

An LRI is performed on all patients who, based on topography readings and the expected SIA, are likely to still have visually significant cylinder. Surgeons who make their incisions superiorly need to be aware that additional against-the-rule cylinder will be induced. For a patient who has 0.50 D of against-the-rule cylinder, it would be appropriate to perform an LRI at 180 degrees preoperatively. Conversely, for a patient who has pre-existing 0.50 D of with-the-rule cylinder, this astigmatism will be corrected by the surgical technique of a superior incision. For oblique astigmatism, a vector analysis of the preoperative astigmatism and incision will yield the correct meridian and magnitude of cylinder to be corrected.

As with any surgical procedure, there are potential complications associated with LRIs, but most are either temporary or correctable. The procedure is generally not associated with glare or starburst, as may be seen with radial keratotomy or AK. The potential problems with LRIs include overcorrection, undercorrection, infection, perforation of the cornea, decreased corneal sensation, induced irregular astigmatism, and discomfort. For patients with significant remaining astigmatism, it may be necessary to retreat the eye by redeepening or extending the LRI. For overcorrections we recommend waiting until the astigmatism is stable, which may take 1 to 2 weeks, and later cleaning out the wound with a Sinskey hook and suturing it with 10-0 nylon, if necessary. For smaller overcorrections, an excimer laser photoablation may be used. We never recommend placing LRIs perpendicular to the original LRIs for consecutive cylinder, as this may induce irregular astigmatism. If the cornea is perforated, it may be self-sealing or a suture may be required.

When a surgeon transitions from "routine" cataract to refractive IOL surgery, it becomes more important to pay attention to detail. One must now be willing and able to address even small

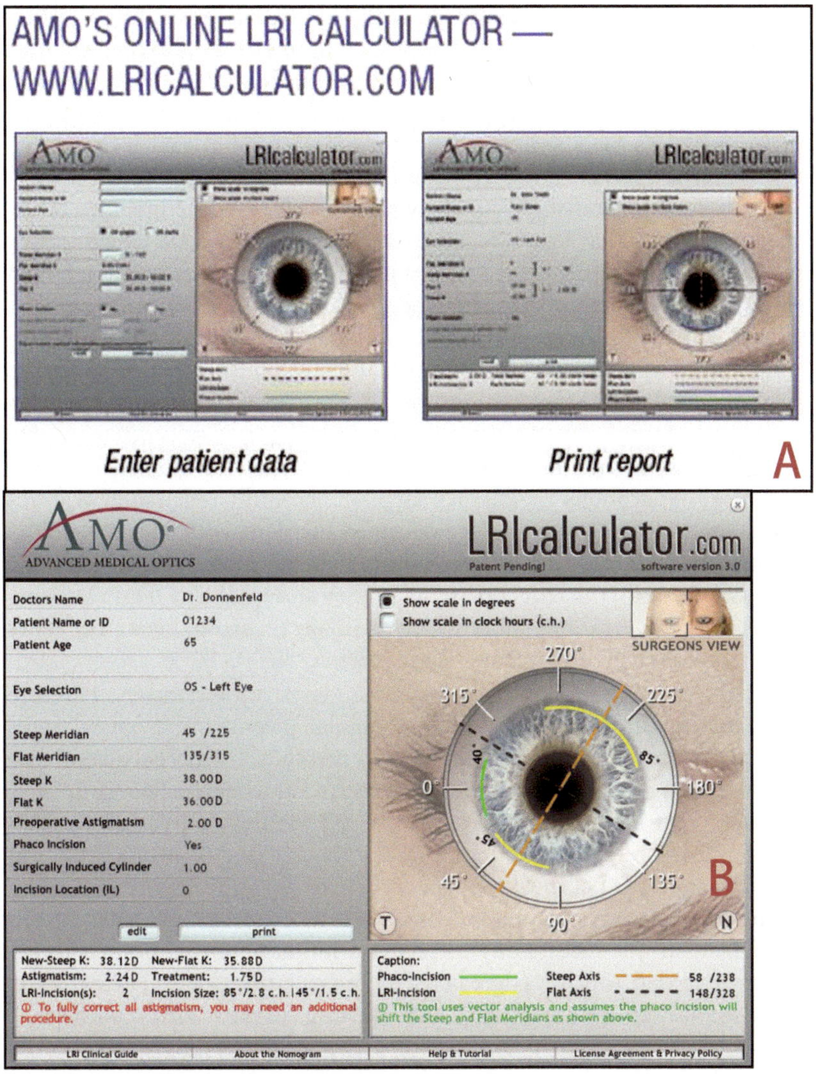

Figure 7-1. (A, B) The Donnenfeld and Nichamin nomogram, available at http://www.LRIcalculator.com.

levels of residual refractive error. Performing LRIs is a major step in this process. Manual LRIs are a forgiving, inexpensive, and repeatable technique that may be performed at the time of implant surgery; they provide rapid visual recovery and do not preclude future excimer laser treatments. However, there can be a variable and unpredictable treatment response due to imprecise depth, length, angulation, and position of the incisions. These concerns, in addition to surgeon variability, make manual LRIs more of an art form than a science.

Femtosecond Laser Technology

Recent developments in femtosecond laser technology have shifted attention from manual LRIs and AK procedures to femtosecond laser-guided surgery. These laser-assisted procedures may offer a greater degree of precision and accuracy than manual methods.[25] The treatment of astigmatism is in fact an integral aspect of this new and emerging field of femtosecond laser-assisted lens surgery, both in regard to patient outcomes and to the financing and reimbursement of surgery.

Femtosecond lasers make use of a photodisruptive process, with extraordinarily short pulse durations of less than 800 femtoseconds (one femtosecond is 10^{-15} seconds). This extremely short pulse duration allows for the cutting of tissue with considerably less energy than the traditional lasers used in ophthalmic surgery. Per-pulse energy can be reduced approximately 1000-fold, from 1^{-10} millijoules for nanosecond lasers (neodymium-doped yttrium aluminum garnet [Nd:YAG]) to 1^{-10} microjoules for femtosecond lasers. These reductions in per-pulse energy result in substantially less collateral tissue damage, shifting from a few millimeters from the intended target for nanosecond lasers to a few microns for femtosecond lasers. Similar to Nd:YAG laser systems, femtosecond laser pulses pass through transparent tissues and can be focused at a predetermined depth.[26] Femtosecond lasers for ophthalmic surgery have been commercially available since 1999. The precision and extremely limited collateral effects of femtosecond pulses on the cornea have been established in more than 4 million procedures performed using femtosecond lasers for the creation of laser in situ keratomileusis (LASIK) flaps as well as lamellar and penetrating keratoplasties.[27-31]

The US Food and Drug Administration has provided 510(k) clearance for the use of several femtosecond lasers for clinical applications in cataract surgery. The most remarkable features of laser cataract surgery include the precision of the performed incisions with minimal collateral damage to surrounding tissues, the accuracy of capsulotomy dimensions and diameters, the enhancement of capsular edge strength, the reduction of phaco power during lens fragmentation, and the improved wound sealing and healing—all of which are likely to lead to better and more reproducible results compared with manual, mechanical surgeries.

As mentioned, a major clinical application of the femtosecond laser is the creation of arcuate incisions that have precise and accurate arc length, depth, angular position, and optical zone, potentially enhancing precision and repeatability over manual methods.[32] One particular case study highlights how the laser can address pre-existing astigmatism during lens-based surgery, in that following the measurement of the patient's refractive and astigmatic error, along with the corneal thickness, the femtosecond laser was used to create the relaxing incisions.[33] Optical coherence tomography (OCT)-controlled corneal pachymetry was performed directly in the area of the intended incisions and then programmed into the laser. The study results showed that with the femtosecond laser, astigmatism was successfully corrected, with an improved best-corrected visual acuity that was better than that which was predicted by preoperative values. Furthermore, the depth and location of the incisions were consistent with the surgical plan. This report serves to confirm that laser technology is able to create uniform corneal incisions precisely and predictably.[33]

Femtosecond lasers appear to be safe in that photodisruption dissipates within 100 μm of the target, providing a substantive margin and distance from Descemet's membrane, thereby avoiding damage to the corneal endothelium and preventing perforation. However, one case has been reported of an inadvertent perforation into the anterior chamber with a femtosecond laser; in this patient, a gas bubble in the anterior chamber alerted the clinician that the incision was not opened, and thus a wound leak was avoided.[34]

In addition, the laser can be programmed to create the main penetrating and side-port incisions, promoting an ideal wound shape for enhanced sealing and healing, with potentially greater reproducibility of induced astigmatism over that of manual keratomes. Early data support this premise for reduced variability, compared with conventional manual incisions.[35] In a study of initial results with the LenSx femtosecond laser (Alcon Surgical), using 9-mm arcuate incisions and a 33% reduction of the Donnenfeld nomogram, a 70% reduction in astigmatism was achieved.[36]

The surgical technique for performing femtosecond laser arcuate incisions first involves determining the length, position, depth, and distance from the visual axis where the incisions will be created. We use a 33% reduction of the Donnenfeld nomogram and use the LRI calculator (www.LRIcalculator.com) to determine the length and axis at which the incision should be placed

Table 7-1. Femtosecond Laser Nomogram

Donnenfeld Nomogram for Manual Limbal Relaxing Incisions		Nomogram for 9 mm Femtosecond Laser Arc Incisions
0.50 D	1 incision, 1 1/2 clock hours (45 degrees each)	1 incision, 1 clock hour (30 degrees each)
0.75 D	2 incisions, 1 clock hour (30 degrees each)	2 incisions, 2/3 clock hours (20 degrees each)
1.50 D	2 incisions, 2 clock hours (60 degrees each)	2 incisions, 1 1/3 clock hours (40 degrees each)
3.00 D	2 incisions, 3 clock hours (90 degrees each)	2 incisions, 2 clock hours (60 degrees each)
*Use 5 degrees more for against-the-rule astigmatism *Use 5 degrees more for younger patients *Use 5 degrees less for older patients		85% depth

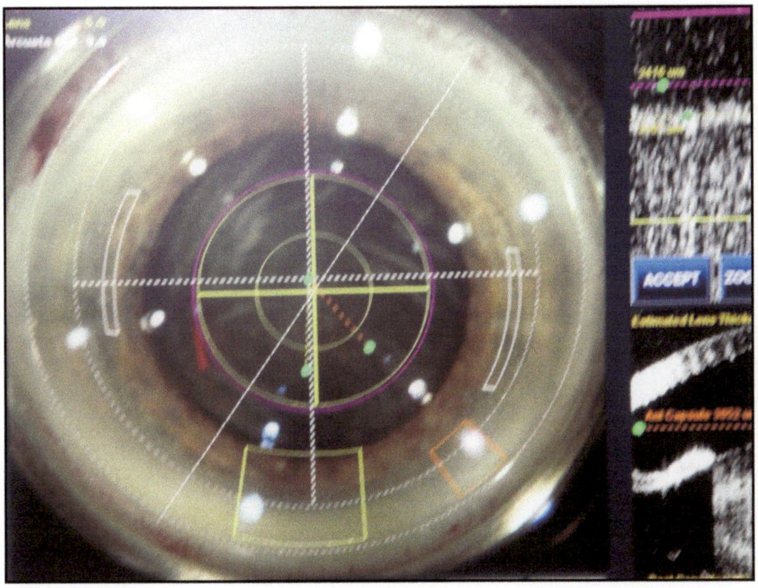

Figure 7-2. Overlay of the arcuate incisions.

(Table 7-1). We preset the depth of our incisions to 85% of the corneal pachymetry in the area of the incision. We also set our distance from the visual axis at 9 mm, and this information is downloaded into the femtosecond laser. We then begin the surgical procedure by docking the laser onto the cornea. An overlay of the incisions is visible on the surgical screen (Figure 7-2). As a safety measure, the corneal and side-port incisions cannot overlap with the astigmatic incision, so there are no intersecting incision planes. Optical coherence tomography imaging of the cornea in the area of the arcuate incision is then visualized, and the depth is confirmed (Figure 7-3). We first perform the capsulotomy, followed by the lens disruption, and then create the corneal incisions. Following completion of the femtosecond laser treatment, the patient is brought to the operating microscope and the incisions are opened with a Sinskey hook (Figure 7-4). Intraoperative aberrometry (ORA; WaveTec Vision) may then be performed to titrate the opening of the incisions. The incisions are symmetric and standardized at 9 mm from the visual

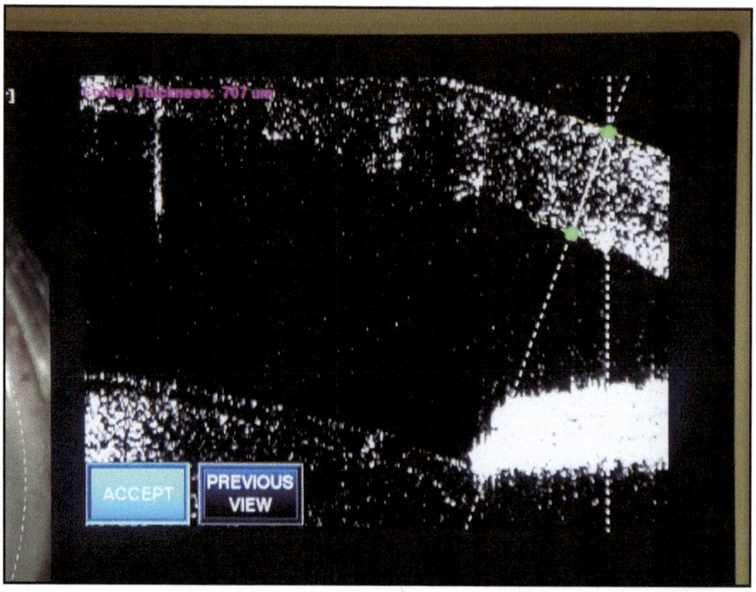

Figure 7-3. OCT imaging of the cornea in the area of the arcuate incision provides precise pachymetry.

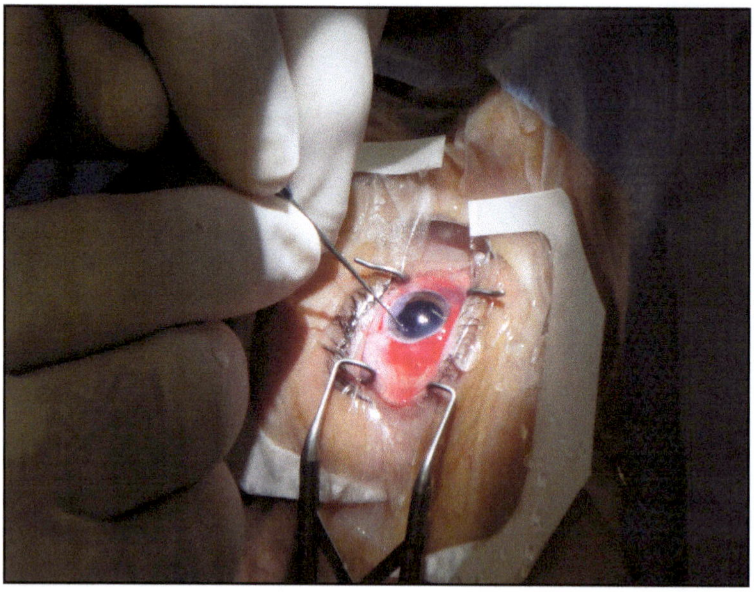

Figure 7-4. Sinskey hook used to open the femtosecond arcuate incisions.

axis (Figure 7-5). Optical coherence tomography confirms the postoperative depth of the incisions (Figure 7-6). If necessary, the arcuate incisions may be further opened postoperatively at the slit lamp using forceps or a Sinskey hook and a topical anesthetic (Figure 7-7).

As femtosecond laser technology emerges, astigmatic relaxing incisions are becoming less of an art form and more of a science, with reproducible arc length, depth, and angulation. In this regard, it is noteworthy that proper angulation may play a role in reducing wound gape, which may be seen with all corneal incisions, but it is more common following incisions to reduce astigmatism. A 135-degree angulation was found to optimally reduce wound gape and improve results.[37] However, although the results have in some cases improved over manual LRIs, there continues to be an unpredictable response to laser-created incisions. This is due to the inherent variable response to corneal incisions, which is based on age, variable thickness, corneal diameter and curvature, intra-

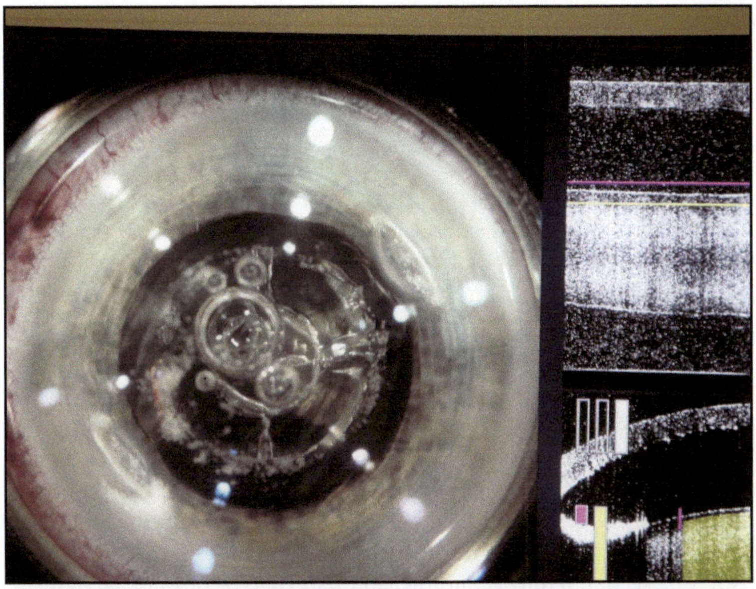

Figure 7-5. Femtosecond arcuate incisions.

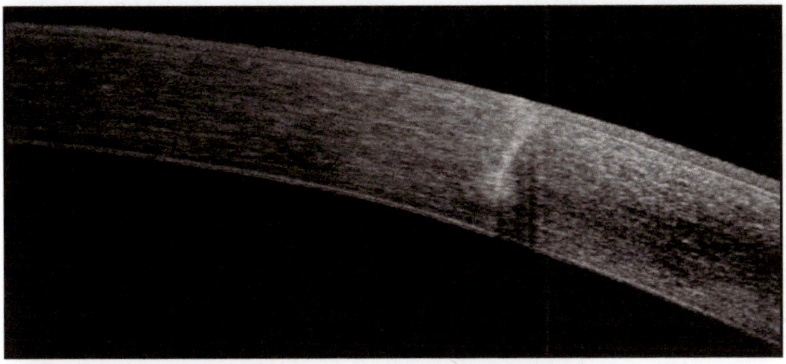

Figure 7-6. OCT demonstrating the depth of the arcuate incision.

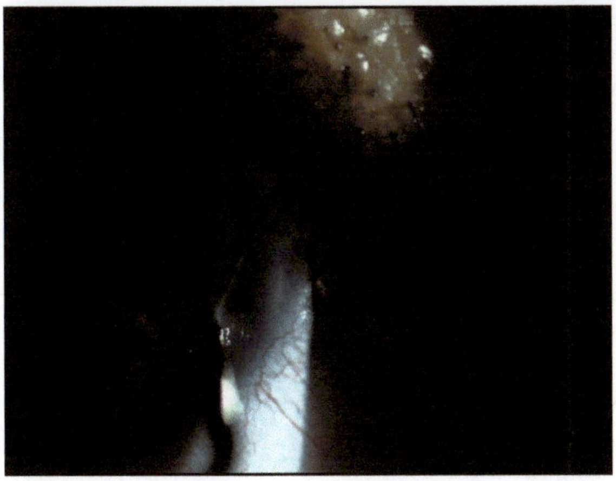

Figure 7-7. Forcep used to open the femtosecond arcuate incision at the slit lamp.

ocular pressure (IOP), and, perhaps most importantly, the biomechanics inherent in the cornea and healing process.

Adjustability of Laser Incisions

A major advantage of femtosecond laser technology is that the refractive incisions may now be made before cataract surgery and then modified intraoperatively and/or postoperatively. When performed with the femtosecond laser, the incisions do not have a full refractive effect until they are opened. We have begun to modify the energy, spot size, and separation of the spots to further refine, titrating our results. With higher energy and small spot size separation, the majority of the effect is achieved without opening the incisions. With lower energy settings and greater spot size separation, the incisions have minimal effect until they are opened. This is the case with femtosecond LASIK flaps because when left in place, they cause no refractive change and essentially disappear until they are opened. A good analogy is that femtosecond laser incisions are similar to a sheet of postage stamps bound together by serrations. Until the serrations are manually torn apart, the stamps remain in a fixed location.

To further refine our results, we have been performing intraoperative aberrometry (ORA), helping to titrate our results in the operating room. We remove the cataract, place the IOL, and open one of the femtosecond laser incisions with a Sinskey hook. The IOP is then raised to approximately 25 mm Hg. We next perform intraoperative aberrometry, which provides an accurate reading of the existing astigmatism. The second femtosecond incision may then be opened partially or completely, based on the intraoperative aberrometry reading, which, if needed, can be taken again. For surgeons who do not have access to intraoperative aberrometry, patients can be examined with topography and refraction performed the day, weeks, or even months after surgery. If needed, the remainder of the incision can be easily opened completely or partially in the desired axis while in the office to increase the effect of the incision and adjust the residual astigmatic refractive error.

In addition to the ability to titrate the LRI with a femtosecond incision, this technology offers a second advantage, which cannot be performed with a manual diamond knife incision; the ability to perform intrastromal sub-Bowman's layer ablations. As noted, these incisions are less powerful than anterior penetrating incisions and may be performed closer to the visual axis. Intrastromal incisions do not cut through Bowman's layer and therefore fewer stromal lamellae are incised, which may provide greater corneal stromal integrity,[36] preserve epithelial integrity,[39,40] reduce pain, and provide a faster recovery. There is no need for postoperative antibiotics because the surface of the eye has not been violated and there may be less likelihood, although long-term results are not available, of late wound drift. Further clinical investigation and nomogram development are currently underway to optimize this method, which would eliminate the need for corneal wound manipulation on the surface.

Conclusion

The creation of femtosecond laser-assisted arcuate incisions is a novel technique that provides the precision of image-guided laser technology. Refractive incisions are now computer-controlled and rely on the surgeon's skill or experience. Our early experience strongly suggests that the use of a femtosecond laser system will provide faster, safer, easier, customizable, adjustable, and fully repeatable astigmatic incisions. In addition, intrastromal ablations may increase the safety and accuracy of astigmatism management. Removing the inconsistencies in the astigmatic procedure will improve our understanding and accuracy of astigmatic incisions and should provide improved refractive results and patient satisfaction. In noting the increased and exciting potential for this technology, we do recognize that further development and refinement of nomograms will be important as surgeons gain and expand their clinical experience.

References

1. Pager CK, McCluskey PJ, Retsas C. Cataract surgery in Australia: a profile of patient-centred outcomes. *Clin Experiment Ophthalmol.* 2004;32(4):388-392.
2. Hawker MJ, Madge SN, Baddeley PA, Perry SR. Refractive expectations of patients having cataract surgery. *J Cataract Refract Surg.* 2005;31(10):1970-1975.
3. Nichamin LD. Nomogram for limbal relaxing incisions. *J Cataract Refract Surg.* 2006;32(9):1048.
4. Ferrer-Blasco T, Montés-Micó R, Peixoto-de-Matos SC, González-Méijome JM, Cerviño A. Prevalence of corneal astigmatism before cataract surgery. *J Cataract Refract Surg.* 2009;35(1):70-75.
5. Hill W. Expected effects of surgically induced astigmatism on AcrySof toric intraocular lens results. *J Cataract Refract Surg.* 2008;34(3):364-367.
6. Duffey RJ, Leaming D. *US trends in refractive surgery: 2008 ISRS/AAO survey.* Paper presented at: International Society of Refractive Surgery & American Academy of Ophthalmology Refractive Surgery Subspecialty Day; November 8, 2008; Atlanta, Georgia.
7. Nichamin LD. Astigmatism control. *Ophthalmol Clin North Am.* 2006;19(4):485-493.
8. Wang L, Misra M, Koch DD. Peripheral corneal relaxing incisions combined with cataract surgery. *J Cataract Refract Surg.* 2003;29(4):712-722.
9. Budak K, Friedman NJ, Koch DD. Limbal relaxing incisions with cataract surgery. *J Cataract Refract Surg.* 1998;24(4):503-508.
10. Gills JP. Treating astigmatism at the time of cataract surgery. *Curr Opinion Ophthalmol.* 2002;13(1):2-6.
11. Oshika T, Shimazaki J, Yoshitomi F, et al. Arcuate keratometry to treat corneal astigmatism after cataract surgery: a prospective evaluation of predictability and effectiveness. *Ophthalmology.* 1998;105(11):2012-2016.
12. Maloney WF, Grindle L, Sanders D, Pearcy D. Astigmatism control for the cataract surgeon: a comprehensive review of surgically tailored astigmatism reduction (STAR). *J Cataract Refract Surg.* 1989;15(1):45-54.
13. Price FW, Grene RB, Marks RG, Gonzales JS; for the ARC-T Study Group. Astigmatism reduction clinical trial: a multicenter prospective evaluation of the predictability of arcuate keratotomy. *Arch Ophthalmol.* 1995;113(3):277-282.
14. Devgan U. Corneal correction of astigmatism during cataract surgery. *Cataract & Refractive Surgery Today.* January 2007:41-44.
15. Tejedor J, Murube J. Choosing the location of corneal incision based on preexisting astigmatism in phacoemulsification. *Am J Ophthalmol.* 2005;139(5):767-776.
16. Kaufmann C, Peter J, Ooi K, Phipps S, Cooper P, Goggin M; for The Queen Elizabeth Astigmatism Study Group. Limbal relaxing incisions versus on-axis incisions to reduce corneal astigmatism at the time of cataract surgery. *J Cataract Refract Surg.* 2005;31(12):2261-2265.
17. Muller-Jensen K, Fischer P, Siepe U. Limbal relaxing incisions to correct astigmatism in clear corneal cataract surgery. *J Refract Surg.* 1999;15(5):586-589.
18. Akura J, Matsuura K, Hatta S, Otsuka K, Kaneda S. A new concept for the correction of astigmatism: full-arc depth-dependent astigmatic keratotomy. *Ophthalmology.* 2000;107(1):95-104.
19. Faktorovich EG, Maloney RK, Price FW Jr. Effect of astigmatic keratotomy on spherical equivalent: results of the Astigmatism Reduction Clinical Trial. *Am J Ophthalmol.* 1999;127(3):260-269.
20. Price FW, Grene RB, Marks RG, Gonzales JS. Astigmatism reduction clinical trial: a multicenter prospective evaluation of the predictability of arcuate keratotomy. Evaluation of surgical nomogram predictability. ARC-T Study Group [published correction appears in *Arch Ophthalmol.* 1995;113(5):577.]. *Arch Ophthalmol.* 1995;113(3):277-282.
21. Bradley MJ, Coombs J, Olson RJ. Analysis of an approach to astigmatism correction during cataract surgery. *Ophthalmologica.* 2006;220(5):311-316.
22. AcrySof Toric SA60T4IOL [package insert]. Fort Worth, TX: Alcon Laboratories Inc.; 2009.
23. Donnenfeld ED, Solomon R. LRIs and Refractive IOLs. In: *Chang, Mastering Refractive IOLs: The Art and Science.* Thorofare, NJ: SLACK Incorporated;2008:601-605.
24. Nichamin LD. Astigmatism control. *Ophthalmol Clin North Am.* 2006;19(4):485-93.
25. Masket S, Sarayba M, Ignacio T, Fram N. Femtosecond laser-assisted cataract incisions: architectural stability and reproducibility. *J Cataract Refract Surg.* 2010;36(6):1048-1049.
26. Vogel A, Noack J, Hüttman G, Paltauf B. Mechanisms of femtosecond laser nanosurgery of cells and tissues. *Appl Phs B.* 2005;81(8):1015-1047.
27. Ratkay-Traub I, Ferincz IE, Juhasz T, Kurtz RM, Krueger RR. First clinical results with the femtosecond neodymium-glass laser in refractive surgery. *J Refract Surg.* 2003;19(2):94-103.
28. Nordan LT, Slade SG, Baker RN, Suarez C, Juhasz T, Kurtz R. Femtosecond laser flap creation for laser in situ keratomileusis: six-month follow-up of initial U.S. clinical series. *J Refract Surg.* 2003;19(1):8-14.
29. Kezirian GM, Stonecipher KG. Comparison of the IntraLase femtosecond laser and mechanical keratomes for laser in situ keratomileusis. *J Cataract Refract Surg.* 2004;30(4):804-811.

30. Montés-Micó R, Rodríquez-Galietero A, Alió JL. Femtosecond laser versus mechanical keratome LASIK for myopia. *Ophthalmology.* 2007;114(1):62-68.
31. Steinert RF, Ignacio TS, Sarayba MA. "Top hat"-shaped penetrating keratoplasty using femtosecond laser. *Am J Ophthalmol.* 2007;143(4):689-691.
32. Nichamin L. Femtosecond laser technology applied to lens-based surgery. *Medscape Ophthalmology.* June 22, 2010. http://www.medscape.com/viewarticle/723864. Accessed July 20, 2011.
33. Nagy Z, Takacs A, Filkom T, Sarayba M. Initial clinical evaluation of an intraocular femtosecond laser in cataract surgery. *J Refract Surg.* 2009;25(12):1053-1060.
34. Vaddavalli PK, Hurmeric V, Yoo SH. Air bubble in anterior chamber as indicator of full-thickness incisions in femtosecond-assisted astigmatic keratotomy. *J Cataract Refract Surg.* 2011;37(9):1723-1725.
35. Abbey A, Ide T, Kymionis GD, Yoo SH. Femtosecond laser-assisted astigmatic keratotomy in naturally occurring high astigmatism. *Br J Ophthalmol.* 2009;93(12):1566-1569.
36. Donnenfeld, ED *Femtosecond laser arcuate incision astigmatism correction in cataract surgery.* Paper presented at: the XXX Congress of the ESCRS; September 8-12, 2012; Milan, Italy.
37. Cleary C, Tang M, Ahmed H, Fox M, Huang D. Beveled Femtosecond laser astigmatic keratotomy for the treatment of high astigmatism post-penetrating keratoplasty. *Cornea.* 2013;32(1):54-62.
38. Binder PS, Gray B, Brownell M, Martiz J, Gown A, Hill J. *Morphology of femtosecond intrastromal arcuate incisions.* Poster presented at: the 2012 ARVO Annual Meeting; May 6-9, 2012; Ft. Lauderdale, FL [2012.03.07-ME4839].
39. Meltendorf C, Burbach GJ, Ohrloff C, Ghebremedhin E, Deller T. Intrastromal keratotomy with femtosecond laser avoids profibrotic TGF-β1 Induction. *Invest Ophthalmol Vis Sci.* 2009;50(8):3688-3695.
40. Rashid ER, Waring III GO. Complications of radial and transverse keratotomy. *Surv Ophthalmol.* 1989;34(2):73-105.

Financial Disclosures

Dr. Noel A. Alpins has financial interest in the ASSORT Surgical Management Systems software program.

Dr. Allon Barsam has not disclosed any relevant financial relationships.

Dr. Eric D. Donnenfeld has financial interest in Alcon Laboratories, Abbott Medical Optics, Bausch & Lomb, and Wavetec Vision.

Dr. James P. Gills has stock ownership in Lenstec.

Dr. Pit Gills has no financial or proprietary interest in the materials presented herein.

Dr. David R. Hardten has no financial or proprietary interest in the materials presented herein.

Dr. Christian C. Hester has no financial or proprietary interest in the materials presented herein.

Dr. Richard S. Hoffman has no financial or proprietary interest in the materials presented herein.

Dr. Douglas D. Koch is a consultant for Alcon Laboratories, Abbott Medical Optics, and Revision Optics; has stock ownership in OptiMedica; and receives research support from i-Optics and Ziemer Ophthalmic Systems.

Dr. Richard L. Lindstrom has not disclosed any relevant financial relationships.

Dr. Molly McDonald has not disclosed any relevant financial relationships.

Dr. Louis D. "Skip" Nichamin is a consultant for Advanced Medical Optics, Allergan, Bausch & Lomb, Foresight Biotherapeutics, Glaukos Corporation, and Liquidia Technologies; an investor in Harvest Precision Components; and a consultant and investor for 3D Vision Systems, eyeonics, iScience Surgical Corporation, LensAR, PowerVision, RevitalVision, and Wavetec Vision Systems. He has no financial interest in any ophthalmic instruments that bear his name.

Dr. Randall J. Olson has no financial or proprietary interest in the materials presented herein.

Dr. Parag D. Parekh has no financial or proprietary interest in the materials presented herein.

Dr. Jonathan B. Rubenstein has not disclosed any relevant financial relationships.

Dr. George Stamatelatos has financial interest in the ASSORT Surgical Management Systems software program.

Dr. Spencer P. Thornton has no financial or proprietary interest in the materials presented herein.

Dr. R. Bruce Wallace III is a consultant for Bausch & Lomb, on the Medical Advisory Board for LensAR, and lectures for Advanced Medical Optics.

Dr. An Vo has no financial or proprietary interest in the materials presented herein.

Index